T0265910

RATTLED

RATTLED

How to Calm New Mom
Anxiety with the Power
of the Postpartum Brain

Nicole Amoyal Pensak, PhD

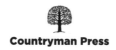

Countryman Press

An Imprint of W. W. Norton & Company
Independent Publishers Since 1923

RATTLED is a general information resource for new mothers. It is not a substitute for individual medical diagnosis or treatment. Every new mother and every new motherhood situation is unique. No one can predict what your experience as a new mother will be. *If you feel severely depressed or you have any doubt or concern about your own physical or emotional health or well-being, consult a mental healthcare professional.* Do not hesitate to seek emergency care for yourself if you think it may be needed.

The patients and their courses of treatment described in this book are composites. Any products that the author recommends in this book are ones that the author personally likes. You need to do your own research to find the products that are best for you.

As of press time, the URLs displayed in this book link or refer to existing websites. The publisher is not responsible for, and should not be deemed to endorse or recommend, any website other than its own or any other content available on the internet or elsewhere, including, without limitation, any app, blog page, or information page that the publisher did not create. The author, also, is not responsible for any third-party material.

For information about permission to reproduce selections from this book, write to Permissions, Countryman Press, 500 Fifth Avenue, New York, NY 10110

For information about special discounts for bulk purchases, please contact W. W. Norton Special Sales at specialsales@wwnorton.com or 800-233-4830

Manufacturing by Lakeside Book Company
Book design by Patrice Sheridan
Production manager: Julia Druskin

Countryman Press
www.countrymanpress.com

An imprint of W. W. Norton & Company, Inc.
500 Fifth Avenue, New York, NY 10110
www.wwnorton.com

978-1-68268-830-4

10 9 8 7 6 5 4 3 2 1

To my incredibly supportive husband, Mike, thank you for building this wonderful life with me.

To Mike, Jordan Vail, and Max Wolf—you have taught me to love more than I could ever imagine. You are endless sources of inspiration and my entire world.

CONTENTS

PART III How to Go from Surviving to Thriving in Early
          Motherhood

INTRODUCTION

"I'm really interested in trying to tell stories about women that don't involve romantic components. There are so many more stories than that." —GRETA GERWIG, DIRECTOR

I paced the floor of my infant son's bedroom, my brain on fire with the typical new mom problems I could not solve. Did Max eat enough during his last feed? Did I need to pump more milk? What if the baby monitor doesn't work and I sleep through a feeding? Was he pleasantly stimulated? Was he *overstimulated*? What if I never slept again?

In the kitchen, I poured myself a second cup of coffee, trying to get my body to catch up to my brain. I felt incapacitated by fear. My mind wasn't working the way it used to. I steadied myself against the counter and tried to force my foggy brain to figure out the answer to *how did I get here?* Me, a clinical psychologist who specializes in anxiety treatment.

I am a certified specialist in perinatal mental health. I work with scores of mothers battling postpartum anxiety and depression. I knew anxiety treatment better than the back of my hand—and had even experienced a version of it with my first child—yet here I was, living through a global trauma while caring for my newborn, paralyzed by my own anxiety. It rattled me to my core. Nine days later, with a diagnosis of postpartum obsessive-compulsive disorder (OCD) and a course of medication and therapy, I began to feel better.

My postpartum experience with Max was different from that of my first child. With Jordan, for months I experienced the normal new mom worries: *Is she eating enough? Is she breathing at night? Is she too hot or cold? How can I prevent her from getting sick?* It was a huge transition to go from worrying about myself to being responsible for keeping a real baby alive. I grappled with the push-pull of early motherhood. I swung back and forth between loving my baby to the moon and back and needing to be *anywhere else* but with my baby. One moment, I'd confidently think, *I got this,* when I remembered to pack the diaper bag with all the things, make it to the doctor's appointment on time, and get a nod of approval from the pediatrician. The next moment? Jordan figured out how to make a corner table safety guard a choking hazard. I'd leap to sweep the recently influenced "item every mom needs to prevent poking injuries" out of her mouth and feel a surge of panic. My heart would drop and I'd think, *I definitely do not have this.*

Biologically, I became a mother overnight. But the psychological adjustment took longer, as did baby bonding and the identity development. My usually put-together, do-it-all persona struggled to navigate common early motherhood realities: new mom worries, forgetfulness and fogginess, hair-trigger temper outbursts, mom rage, mood swings, guilt and shame, challenges with breastfeeding, and ambivalence. All of it rattled me.

With both babies, however, I was able harness the seismic changes in motherhood and land in a place I didn't anticipate: better than ever. In this book, and as soon as you see those two pink lines on the pee stick, I want to share with you how.

Though I'm a psychologist, I was not immune to postpartum anxiety. It didn't matter that I was trained at Harvard and Yale, nor was it relevant that I specialized in the exact thing I would be diagnosed with. Academic training and longtime work with patients didn't mean a thing since I had never been a mother. My postpartum anxiety revealed itself after both of my children were born, the second time with a vengeance. My own experience with anxiety gave me personal insight, guided by my understanding of maternal brain neuroplasticity processes, evidence-based mental health treatment, and my knowledge of the transformation of becoming a mother, known as matrescence, I was able to climb out of rock bottom. With the perfect vision of hindsight, I know we can absolutely do better to prepare mothers for the transition—biological and psychological, earth-shattering and amazing—into motherhood. We are in this together.

Mothers need to know what they are working with under the hood: maternal brain changes, normal mom worries that are adaptive, worries that are not helpful, and how to harness it all, backed by science and therapy. When you become a mother, the biological process moves fast, while the psychological process lags behind. When we are used to functioning at a high level, these two out-of-sync processes take us by surprise. By understanding both the physiological and the psychological, we can make clear-eyed decisions to nurture the process of matrescence. We can learn to accept what is typical: ambivalence, mom worries, interruptions, forgetfulness, unexpected thoughts, postpartum pressures, and new emotions. We can harness both the struggles and the gifts that motherhood provides. As new mothers, we can thrive.

I landed in a place I couldn't have predicted: feeling and functioning at my best. But it was hard work. It is difficult to make use of maternal gifts when we are in the trenches, bogged down by the challenges of modern motherhood. Throughout this book, I will share how to tap into your maternal power. I will teach you how to remove common roadblocks that prevent you from reaching your full potential. Throughout, I'll provide tools to new families to distinguish what is going on, what is physiological, and what is psychological. And I will elucidate the common postpartum experiences, why problems like postpartum depression go underdiagnosed and undertreated, and how to nurture your maternal mental health.

There is no better time than now to focus on maternal mental health. Coming out of a global pandemic, the United States is currently undergoing a maternal mental health crisis. But let's face it: moms have *always* fought the internal currents working against them. Recent research suggests that mothers undergo a transformation of neuroplasticity in the brain, both physiologically induced and experience dependent.[1] The maternal brain endures a structural and cellular remodeling unlike any other discrete period in human development and continues to reorganize itself and evolve based on mothers' experiences with the infant.[2] But many of these biological and hormone-driven "neuroplastic" changes that are beneficial to the baby can be simultaneously deleterious to the mother. Turns out, there is good reason for that. Pregnant women have vulnerable immune systems because the mother's immune system is working to protect the developing baby in the womb.[3] This means that mothers are more susceptible to getting sick and developing infections. Hormonal changes that promote baby's fetal development can lead to increased vulnerability for mental health conditions for the mother.[4] To sum it up, the same brain changes that evolve to make you a good mom to your baby can work against your own mental health.

While mothers provide a valuable boost to their babies' immune systems and protect their infants from infection, they sacrifice their own mental health because these physiological changes are associated with mental health conditions, including postpartum depression and anxiety (PPDA). Postpartum depression is the most common complication associated with childbirth. Prior to the pandemic, it was once estimated to impact between 10 and 20 percent of women.[5] Post-pandemic, the maternal rate for postpartum depression is as high as one in three mothers.[6] For postpartum anxiety, the rates are 26 percent but are underdiagnosed and undertreated.[7] The pandemic was a global trauma, especially for mothers. It is reported that first-time mothers during the pandemic are now having their second babies, and because they could not process what was going on during the pandemic, the unprocessed trauma is now retriggering and retraumatizing these second-time mothers. Mothers are still afraid of reporting their symptoms because they are afraid they will be viewed as "unfit." Further research suggests that the accurate rates of perinatal mental health conditions are as high as 72 percent since the pandemic. If you consider yourself a "supermom"—the high-functioning type who wants to do it all and has perfectionistic tendencies (aka wanting to make the best, most informed decisions, hence why you are also reading this book)—the most current research states you are at an even greater risk for postpartum anxiety.[8]

While this book focuses on biological mothers and primary caregivers, the strategies and guidance provided can also benefit nonbiological caregivers and LGBTQ parents. The most recent research suggests that sexual minority parents are not at an increased risk for developing perinatal mood disorders, contrary to prior research that suggested they were.[9] However, they are still at a similar risk compared to heterosexual and biological parents, which is significant.

I will not provide a checklist of symptoms of perinatal depression and anxiety for you to self-assess. I think that is part of the problem with modern-day motherhood. I give you a list of symptoms and you self-assess, self-monitor, find a therapist, schedule an appointment, etc. There are many things you will need to do to take care of your mental health—diagnosing yourself should not be one of them. All you need to feel is that something is off, you don't feel like yourself, that you're not enjoying this as much as you think you could or should. Make an appointment to talk with a provider and go from there. Let the doctors do their jobs. You have enough to do.

Besides the physiological and environmental difficulties that work against new mothers, there is a lot of good news that is not often shared with mothers. With new motherhood, this heightened period of neuroplasticity brings with it opportunities and risk. The opportunities are now starting to gain attention. Recent research suggests that changes in mothers' brains regarding reward and motivation result in increased sensitivity when responding to their own babies, heightened fear reactivity, and some decreases in memory functioning (a component of "mommy brain").[10] In fact, functional magnetic resonance imaging (fMRI) studies confirm that some of these processes are correlated with a more adaptive attachment with the baby.[11] Beyond that, most recent research extends neuroplasticity to highlight the ways motherhood benefits the brain. Indeed, pregnant women experience boosts in cognitive abilities related to child-rearing. Mothers, compared to nonmothers, demonstrate better emotion regulation, flexibility, and abilities related to social cognition, empathy, and mentalization.[12] Visual memory abilities are also improved in both mothers and fathers.

The truth about mommy brain is also coming to light with emerging recognition of its brilliance. No longer will the mommy brain be branded as a dysfunction or deficit characterized by fogginess and forgetfulness. While mothers subjectively experience these problems, research showing meaningful memory deficits are sparse. Instead, we need to understand the full capabilities of maternal brain power, above and beyond the up-until-now narrow and limited scope. Here, you will discover what your incredible mommy brain has to offer. The good news is that new mothers might also surf this tidal wave of neuroplasticity, the brain's ability to change and reorganize itself, developing into the better-than-ever brain I eventually found.[13] Research is still in its infancy, and there has yet to be an intervention to specifically promote plasticity in an adaptive way for new mothers. But I am hopeful that, in time, there will be. This book moves the conversation forward.

How to Use This Book

Parents, friends, even strangers in a grocery store tell you, "You'll miss these days when they're out of the house." They tell you to "enjoy every moment!" But no one tells you how exactly to enjoy every single moment while you just got through aisle two of the grocery store and can smell *and see* the blowout from your baby's diaper. How exactly do you enjoy each moment when you are up at 4 AM with a colicky baby? Wiping spit-up from your shirt for the 20th time? Feeling something crunchy in your hair during a new client meeting—oatmeal from the breakfast your baby flung at you or maybe from the midnight snack you inhaled after the baby woke? You'll wash it out—whenever you manage to shower.

How do you love every moment when you haven't had a hot dinner in weeks or when you stubbed your toe in the dark on the way to get your crying baby for her 2 AM feeding? When your baby is an early riser and your toddler burns the midnight oil? It's especially challenging to enjoy moments with your partner. He's explaining his big meeting the next day, but you are mentally making a list of the doctor appointments you need to schedule, groceries you need to pick up, laundry you need to finish, and participation forms and waivers you need to fill out for *all the things*. The mental load of motherhood is overwhelming.

Enjoying the early days is a challenge when your postpartum brain worries about the baby breathing at night. Or about the consistency of the poop in his diaper, exposure to illness before immunizations, providing enough stimulation, or starting him on solid foods too early or too late. All while working through the unanticipated challenges of breastfeeding or formula dietary issues. *This is not what you expected.*

But those strangers insist that you enjoy every moment, and so, early on in motherhood, I tried to do that. I loved looking at those big blue globes staring back at me, reflecting everything that matters. I loved grazing her soft skin and squishy, slightly pink cheeks. I tried, I really tried, to love through every minute of every day. And just when I thought my heart would explode because I couldn't possibly love anything more, I encountered a sleep regression that left me up all night, another weird rash that needed a doctor appointment, a nap schedule that prevented us from a fun event, or a bout of the stomach bug brought home from her first weeks at daycare. I tried my best to be calm, to be patient with the relentlessness of it all, but the sleepless nights, rotating illnesses, and regressions sometimes got the best of me.

That urge to yell, or slam a door, or run, goes from 0 to 100 in seconds. I felt terrible for wanting an escape, and I immediately recommitted to be a cycle breaker. I, like many, was raised by parents born in a generation of behaviorists. Compliance was the goal. I committed and envisioned that I would do things differently. So I wanted to start right out of the gate adhering to impossible mothering standards—being an endless resource of patience, love, and empathy while singing soft and soothing lullabies as I relentlessly tended to my baby.

The mom guilt set in and I thought, *I should not be feeling this way.* I knew I *would* miss these moments. I fast-forwarded to seeing her off to college. Some tears welled up. I must be doing something wrong. I must not be maternal. Mothering is so much *easier* for everyone else.

One day I realized that, somewhere along the line, mothers need to understand the specific, momentous birth of a mother and transition to motherhood. We need to educate moms on what to really expect for themselves, their role transition, and the complete overhaul of their brain and psyche. This book is the answer to how to better equip mothers.

My realization led to this book. In these pages, I answer the questions that I asked myself: How can we better support the mother in early motherhood? Perinatal visits focus on the fetus and then the physical clearance of the birthing parent, but who holds the caregiver? How is the mother supposed to adjust to the very real brain and identity changes that occur in early motherhood with no education about how her new maternal brain functions? How are new mothers supposed to figure out what is important to worry about and what's not?

This book will teach you to manage new mom worries, understand biological and psychological brain changes, and create a foolproof postpartum plan. I share evidence-based strategies for managing mental health and how to handle a perinatal mental health crisis. You will learn to use brain plasticity to your advantage in early motherhood. I discuss how to manage mom guilt, mom shame, and mom rage, as well as the role identity transformation to motherhood. I dispel the common caregiver myth that a mother has to sacrifice her own well-being for the benefit of her child. I will show you how to break the cycle of unmet needs, understand your newfound pleasure, and cultivate and integrate creativity into being a primary caregiver. This book will teach you how to go from rattled to rocking it in early motherhood.

I will teach you how to recognize high-functioning depression and anxiety, and suggest you get help and don't try to diagnose and treat yourself. I will educate you on the nuances of these conditions. Mothers are expected to do it all and somehow just adapt. When doubt, frustration, fear, and struggle arise, mothers think they are failing. When mothers feel overwhelmed, hopeless, down, and unable to bond or enjoy early motherhood, they turn inward, looking to themselves to blame. When they worry or experience challenges that feel impossible, they think they are doing it wrong. Instead of fully understanding and appreciating the gravity of the role and transition, they pick up bits and pieces of parenting techniques, false "self-care," and maladaptive coping mechanisms. These are Band-Aids. I will show you the momentous transformation of becoming a mother, the potential pitfalls, and how to nurture the transition and promote healing and strength.

When we label the process, the mechanisms of action and their characteristics, we understand what is happening and can make informed, deliberate decisions. I have patients tell me that it helps them to know when they are "pruning"—getting rid of negative thoughts and beliefs that are no longer serving them in early motherhood, and envisioning their brain getting rid of neural networks they don't need. By identifying the endless cycles of worry, self-criticism, guilt, and shame, we can more accurately pinpoint what is happening instead of getting lost trying to feel our way through.

Rattled is a call-to-action book. It empowers mothers to find support and proper mental health care, to nurture themselves separate from their child's needs, and to understand that *this* is optimal for the child's development. This book focuses on the primary parent or caregiver, with the premise that the majority of motherhood is really managing your own emotions and well-being. Key to this premise is the science of neuroplasticity and cognitive behavioral therapy. Untangling and making new pathways in your brain and increasing psychological flexibility is like getting that knot out of your fine-strand necklace.

This book will help you understand your maternal brain and apply science-based strategies to go from bonkers to brilliant. First, we mothers must accept that motherhood is *impossible*. But navigating the impossible is what this book is about.

Before the first chapter begins, I want to share another important idea. Most of the early parenthood books focus on the child and what is going on inside them. The secret is that a significant portion of taking care of babies involves regulating your own emotions first. You can fuel up your tank and get into prime shape to head out on the one-way highway that is motherhood. I am not saying classic parenting books aren't helpful. They very well can be! You will always have to do a ton of parenting. I am suggesting that educating and encouraging mothers to use their newly developed and very real changed parent brains to their advantage will be life-changing. I can help you get out of your own way and teach you how to drive that souped-up sports car on the highway at full speed. Sure, there may be roadblocks, construction, storms, and accidents along the way, but you'll be better equipped and more able to see what the actual barriers are and how to problem-solve more effectively. Further, you'll be able to see more clearly because your internal system won't interfere with your vision. You'll be able to more optimally perform and function as a mother.

Each chapter includes personal narrative, clinical case examples, or stories that demonstrate the theme of the chapter. Science is integrated throughout, including research studies, facts, and support for the theme. Practical strategies are offered as ways to apply the knowledge from the chapter to your daily life. Each chapter includes Snapshot boxes—brief takeaways that you can review for quick reference.

To use this book, create a new photo album in your phone. Go ahead, do it now. You can title it whatever you would like. It can simply be called "RATTLED," "My Mom Manual," "Sh*#storm Instructions," or even "F&@! This is Hard!" Whatever you decide to call the album of strategies, your guide will be neatly organized and ready in the palm of your hand. Take pictures of the Snapshot boxes you see in each chapter. Since one of the most common experiences in motherhood is being interrupted, the Snapshot boxes are brief summaries with key points. At the end, voilà! Your easy access guide will be available to review as it sits on your nightstand, during those middle-of-the-night feedings, in the bathroom, on a family trip, while you're taking your baby for a walk in the stroller, or while you're hiding in the pantry, eating cookies. There is no need to try to memorize the guide because it is always with you. In this way, I will be with you as a companion, a thought partner, a guide through this incredible opportunity to become the parent you want to be, the mother you never had, the mother you always imagined, and the mother you never even dreamed of becoming. You will become the thriving mother.

PART I

How to Really Prepare for Motherhood

1

THE IDEAL MOTHER

"When you have a baby, you're going to meet an entirely new person: you."   —AUTHOR UNKNOWN

Among the many revelations I expected to experience in early motherhood, being fascinated by octopuses was not one of them. Nor did I expect to learn so much from Netflix.

"Can we watch that again?" I asked my husband. *My Octopus Teacher* had finished. I turned to see that he had fallen asleep and, from the sound of his whisper snore, he had likely been asleep for the latter half of the documentary. I made a note to respond with tonight's incident when he accused me of sleeping through another episode of *Mountain Men*. I reached for my laptop under the right side of my bed and typed, "What is the plural term for octopus?" If I am going to start talking to people about my newfound fascination, I should know the correct plural phrase. Is it octopus? Octopi? Octopuses? Come to find out the correct term is octopuses. If I teach you nothing else in this book, I have at least taught you the correct plural term for octopus.

Down I plunged into the internet abyss of octopus articles. Titles such as "The World's Best Mother" and "The Hardest Working Mom on the Planet" came up. I was intrigued—the octopus is the world's greatest mother? Perhaps it is their ability to quickly adapt to the challenges of their environment, something we are constantly trying to master as mothers of infants. Perhaps it is their unique ability to camouflage that protects their babies from aggressive predators. But it's probably because of their eight arms. An octopus could rock a baby, tightly fasten a swaddle, cook dinner, dry her hair, call the pediatrician, change the Diaper Genie bag, and fold the laundry with each of her eight mother octopus arms. If I had eight arms, I would be the world's best mother too.

I read on. I learn that mother octopus has 10,000 to 200,000 babies and broods on top of those eggs for up to 4½ years. It is during this time that the mother octopus does not leave to eat, gather food, swim, or socialize. She does nothing else but tend to her baby octopus eggs. During the 4½ years, she undergoes a process known as the "death spiral," withering away to a corpse of herself, slowly losing all her brilliant color, her energy, her vibrancy. And once those babies hatch, she kills herself. That's right—she offs herself as soon as her octopus babies are born.

This is the *world's best mother?!* I gawked. How is this exemplary for motherhood? She literally ends her life the day her cephalopod babies are born! The authors of the aforementioned articles, Jeremy Hance and Robert Krulwich, both cite biologist Jim Cosgrove's lecture titled "No Mother Could Give More." As I read their names, something told me that they have no firsthand experience with motherhood.

It dawned on me that yes, this is *exactly* what our society expects of mothers and *everything* that is wrong with the notion of motherhood. In some sort of twisted trade-off, there is an unspoken mother martyrdom culture out there—an invisible competition of who can do more for their babies and the least for themselves. The greater the sacrifice, the better the mother. As a clinical psychologist who treats patients suffering with anxiety and depression every day, I can tell you that it's no wonder that the octopus mother marches down a death spiral after neglecting *every single one* of her own needs for 4½ years. I'm no octopus expert, but from my human perspective I can attest that if I were to do nothing else but lay on top of my 10,000 to 200,000 baby octopus eggs for 53 months, I would lose the will to live too. We humans are also at risk of this when we neglect our own needs to the point of becoming depressed, overwhelmed, and anxious.

The transition to motherhood is the single greatest transformation a person's body will go through in the shortest period. The many profound biological changes that occur to prepare a woman's body for motherhood parallel the early octopus's experience. First, pregnant women have weakened immune systems, giving up their resources to boost the baby's fetal development. Hormonal changes also important for a baby's development in the womb make a mother more vulnerable to postpartum mental health conditions. Due to maternal brain changes, mothers are more attuned to responding to their own babies, as well as experiencing increased fear, and feeling foggy and forgetful (aka "mommy brain."). Yes, mommy brain is a very real phenomenon that occurs due to actual structural brain changes and changes in neurotransmitter activity pre- and postpartum. In simple terms, your brain is working against you, compelling you to ignore your own needs and instead attune to your baby's.

In a recent study examining early motherhood experiences, new moms' most common responses were worrying, fogginess and forgetfulness, and being interrupted.[14] Where do all those lost mom-brain thoughts go? I am convinced that they all escape to some black hole that swallows them up and they never appear again. Wouldn't it be something if they could all get together in some kind of encyclopedia moms could revisit after they nurture their transition and their brains are more fine-tuned as a result? I imagine that, in addition to forgetting the little things like what you ate for dinner last night, big insights are gone too—maybe even flashes of clarity that could solve some foreign crises. They got away from some mom who was just overtired from waking up to baby cries five times the night before. In any case, these maternal brain changes don't help mommies save the world; they simply help them attend to their infant.

It's time to rebrand "mommy brain." A recent article published in *JAMA Neurology* by neuroscientist and maternal brain expert Dr. Jodi Pawluski advises that mothers should be educated about the real brain changes that occur in early motherhood.[15] It is also important to dispel the myth of mommy brain only being negative, a deficit, and dysfunction. In her own research, pregnant women reported the commonly experienced forgetfulness. However, when memory was actually tested in the experiments with baby-related tasks, memory functioning was improved and actually represented a "boost in learning." Furthermore, pregnant women compared to nonpregnant women demonstrated better long-term memory overall. Pawluski also astutely points out that one of the reasons that the negative connotation associated with the mommy brain label is that society expects mothers to be perfect. Thus, any mistake, lapse in memory, or momentary forgetfulness is seen as a problem. If the same forgetfulness was demonstrated by a non-mother, though, perhaps it would go unnoticed. Furthermore, a mother is tasked with an immense mental load while caregiving under stressful conditions (e.g., distraction and interruptions by baby-related demands, an ongoing checklist of various needs to meet, as well as anxiety, depression, physical discomfort, and sleep deprivation from breasts that are engorged and need to be expressed), which could impact the ability to concentrate.

A recent and exciting study investigating the adaptations of the maternal brain at one year postpartum compared 40 non-mothers to mothers who were similar in age and education.[16] The study was the first of its kind to show increased brain activity in the regions of the brain associated with maternal parenting at rest and while not engaged in a baby-related task. These six regions are collectively known as the "caregiver network" and are associated in other studies with post-partum depression, maternal caregiving, and cognition. Results also showed that the mothers, compared to non-mothers, scored higher on tasks that were designed to measure social cognition—how our brains process social information to make sense of the world and people in it. This includes the ability to understand other peoples' emotions, thoughts, and beliefs and that they may be separate from their own. In addition, mothers who performed better on problem-solving tasks demonstrated increased abilities in "cognitive efficiency"—the ability to think, learn, and remember things more easily and effectively. Mothers had "a more responsive, flexible, and efficient emotion-regulation system" compared to their non-mother counterparts. Mothers also reported higher levels of sleep dysfunction, anxiety, and depression. Despite these differences in well-being, mothers still demonstrated advantages in performance.

SNAPSHOT

The Ideal Mother

- The maternal human brain goes through a structural and cellular remodeling to reorganize and evolve based on the mother's experiences with her infant.
- Some neuroplastic changes that are good for the baby can work against the mother.
- The same brain changes that make mothers more responsive and more attuned to babies' needs can work against mothers' mental health.
- The greater the hormonal changes during the postpartum period, the more protective a mother feels toward the child, but at greater risk to the mother's mental health.
- Recent studies point to some cognitive benefits in mommy brain, including boosts in baby-related learning, memory, task performance, social cognition, and cognitive efficiency, and more flexible and efficient emotion-regulation systems.

In a similar vein, a promising article published by Edwina Orchard and colleagues at the Yale Child Study Center at the Yale School of Medicine was published in *Trends in Cognitive Sciences* in January 2023, calling for redefining matrescence as its own neurocognitive developmental stage.[17] The article explains that the significant brain changes during this phase, combined with the "mental load" of motherhood, force mothers to adapt to their heightened responsibilities. In this way, they are faced with incredible and numerous challenges during an opportune time to learn. Their brain continues to fine-tune itself while rising to each new challenge and, as a result, it has the potential to increase cognitive reserve in the long term. Cognitive reserve is defined as the brain's capacity to handle impairment due to illness, loss, and decline over time. The researchers illustrate a model whereby the mother benefits from the experience of managing complexity throughout her lifetime and potentially may exhibit neurological benefits in terms of cognitive reserve. This book is designed to fine-tune mothers' abilities to manage the complexities of the challenges of motherhood in more nuanced ways, in the end becoming better than ever.

SNAPSHOT

The Ideal Mother

- Cutting-edge research advocates for matrescence to be understood as a neurocognitive developmental stage.
- The transition to motherhood is the single greatest physiological transformation a person's body will go through in the shortest period of time.
- When you become a mother, you are physically and psychologically a different person.

When I spoke to another expert in maternal mental health research, Helena Rutherford, PhD, director of The Before and After Baby Lab at Yale School of Medicine, I asked her if she could tell every expecting and new mother one thing about their brain, what would she want them to know? She said, "When we speak about development, the conversation usually ends at adulthood. However, what we know now is that the transition to motherhood is prolific in terms of neural development. This transformation serves as an opportunity for intervention where we can leverage plasticity to improve maternal mental health care."

The observations of the maternal brain have the potential to profoundly impact mothers. Decades of cultural suppression of mothers may finally be shifting to tell the full truth about the brilliance of mommy brain. More research should examine the maternal brain. This would ideally include maternal brain mapping, developing and testing interventions with focus groups, and qualitative interviews; followed by pilot randomized controlled trials; then full-scale randomized controlled trials to show efficacy; and finally, "real-world" effectiveness randomized controlled trials. This series of well-established research steps would yield "evidence" to better understand the maternal brain. I have faith that programs of research will get there and the brilliance of mommy brain will be well established by the time I am old and gray. In the meantime, this book will advance the conversation, share the research we have to date, and adapt the science so mothers can get a head start on current trends in academic research. Mothers need this information now.

The Ideal Mother

- Decades of research show underwhelming evidence differences in memory functioning, aka "mommy brain," despite mothers' subjective reports of forgetfulness, lapses in memory, and fogginess. The picture is incomplete.
- Academic research is moving in the direction of understanding the brilliance of mommy brain and providing a more complete picture.
- Societal pressure to be the "ideal mom" and the suppression of women have facilitated the acceptance of the stereotyped mommy brain as dysfunctional.
- The maternal brain is brilliant, a fact that is backed by decades of research.

In addition to the physiological, it is imperative to nurture your psychological growth as a mother. The shocking identity transformation of becoming a mother is pervasive. Mom blogs, Instagram memes, parenting articles, TikTok videos . . . social media accounts are flooded with bite-sized chunks of mothers everywhere sharing their humorous anecdotes of becoming a mom. The memes attempt to normalize commonalities, including complicated feelings such as going back to work, wanting more "me" time, plopping babies in front of *Cocomelon* for a psychological break, promoting the Fed Is Best campaign referring to both breastmilk and formula being equally great sources of food for babies, and doing "less." Moms who share their vulnerabilities and compassion for themselves are being praised. The once-silent moms who stewed in their own shame for not feeling adequate are finding their voices, realizing that *every other mom* feels the same way. Moms are rattled by motherhood. There is no world's greatest mother.

Every mother wants permission and validation for her choices, and most mothers inherently want to do their best. The problem is that as a society we have increasingly looked for more answers, more strategies, more consumerism to perfect taking care of babies. With the best intentions, mothers have evolved as a culture to rely on external "solutions" instead of cultivating their own brilliance. Mothers seek out more information, more answers, more fixed ways of doing things, more baby bento boxes, and that in turn has exacerbated anxiety in moms and contributed to a vicious cycle of checking and needing to check more. As a culture, we have access to more information than ever before. In the world of social media, everyone can have a page, a voice, advice, and information to help take better care of a baby.

Think about it. In your best moments, you are managing your emotions to be present. Then you can think how to problem-solve, sit with difficult emotions, and tend to your baby's needs because you can understand what they are by seeing beyond yourself. There are scientific justifications as to how this works, and I will share them with you. This book is a prescription—doctor's orders for mothers to fill their cup, with unlimited refills to take care of themselves. You simply cannot serve from an empty vessel.

Here's some more good news. If you are struggling in early motherhood, this is the opportunity for you to come out better than before. If you have complicated feelings about becoming a mother, perhaps from your experience with your own mother, a traumatic birth experience, struggle with anxiety or depression, or you're just finding motherhood incredibly challenging and want to do better, you will. In the psychology world, there is an optimal stress curve where we perform best with some level of stress. Not too much or we become overwhelmed, and not too little or we are undermotivated. The same is true for early motherhood.

Furthermore, there is another phenomenon in psychology called post-traumatic growth (PTG). PTG refers to becoming even more resilient and better than ever as a result of traumatic experience. It may not seem like it, but trauma is a common experience in mother-hood. It is estimated that 3 to 16 percent of mothers experience birth trauma. More commonly, many women find the experience of child-birth emotionally traumatic. Not to mention that becoming a mother is its own "trauma." The late Ralph Hoffman, professor of psychia-try at Yale School of Medicine, described motherhood as a normative trauma. Trauma is, by definition, a deeply distressing experience. The word implies something out of the norm. Normative is establishing, relating to, or deriving from a standard or norm, especially of behav-ior. What is more distressing than giving birth? Yet women have been having babies since the dawn of time. There is no greater normative behavior except death, its equal. In recent history, the pandemic was a global trauma in which most moms were suffering. The mothers who were able to make meaning, find the silver linings, and find ways to make the pandemic work to their advantage—becoming better than ever—are examples of PTG, myself included.

Studies suggest that PTG occurs following 10 percent to 77 per-cent of traumatic events.[18] PTG can only happen when the mother is supported enough to use the "gifts" from the trauma to make positive changes. Often PTG can reveal improved relationships with others, an enhanced appreciation for life, heightened meaning and purpose, new paths in life, and increased personal resilience and strength. If trauma leads to depression, anxiety, post-traumatic stress disorder (PTSD), and other negative outcomes, then we miss out on the opportunity to become an enhanced version of ourselves through this opportunity for growth. Many mothers have this incredible prospect for PTG, both originating from a distressing place and from the normative place of becoming a mother.

Mothers who struggle ask the challenging questions. We dig deep to heal what we thought never could be healed. For many, mother-hood is the motivation to do better. It is the ultimate catalyst to help you improve yourself because the reward is to enjoy one of life's most amazing gifts more fully and benefit the next generation. Is anything else more important? You can reach new heights of thriving through the vectors of early motherhood struggles. You just have to understand, work through each success by building on the previous one, and gain mastery.

It's time to remove the obstacles that are in your way. It's time to thrive.

SNAPSHOT

The Ideal Mother

- Say goodbye to that pre-mom version of yourself, grieve, and mourn the loss of that person.
- Accept that this will be a journey, a discovery of a more enhanced version of yourself through motherhood.
- This book will teach you how to use brain changes to your advantage.
- If you are struggling in motherhood, like many, this is an opportunity for you to come out better than before.
- Becoming a mother is a type of "normative" trauma.
- Even in the worst conditions—traumatic birth, postpartum mental health conditions, and an unhealed mother wound—a phenomenon called post-traumatic growth can allow you to become better than ever.
- Motherhood can be the ultimate motivation to do better. You can learn how to harness that energy and direct it to your advantage to thrive.

2

THE REAL MOMMY BRAIN

"When society wants to focus on 'getting our bodies back,' potty-training from birth, and getting back to work, more focus should be placed on how the maternal brain is setting you up for motherhood and its brilliance."
—BRIDGET CALLAGHAN, PHD, CLINICAL PSYCHOLOGIST AND
DIRECTOR OF THE BRAIN AND BODY LAB AT UCLA

"I can't remember anything. My brain has gone to mush!" Heidi exclaimed as she sat in her chair for session. I listened intently and gestured for her to explain more. She described the all-too-familiar challenges of trying to maintain an adult conversation with her friends, remembering her to-do list in the early weeks of returning to work, and recalling household chores that needed to be completed. "I don't understand, I used to remember everything. I never had to write things down before. Now I walk into a room and forget what I intended to do. I had to retrace my steps just this morning and then just gave up because it took too long to try to figure it out. I also forget so many things at work."

As I looked at the high-powered attorney sitting across from me, I could see she was disappointed in herself, feeling like there was something wrong with her. I paused to see if I could guide her to a more compassionate place. "How are things going with Eliza?" I asked about her four-month-old baby. "Things are going well. I seem to keep everything straight with her—the feedings, the doctor appointments, the necessities . . . we never seem to run out of diapers or wipes," she said, noting that she always remembers to place the Amazon orders.

I can't tell you how many times a new mom has showed up for session thinking there is something wrong with her because her brain isn't functioning in the same ways that it used to. I explained to Heidi—and side note, I am thinking about having this recording playing in the waiting room of my office—"I hear your frustrations and feeling disappointed in yourself. That's a painful feeling. The brain changes in many ways postpartum, and lapses in memory are very common. The good news is that your brain is actually not functioning in an objectively worse way, even though it feels that way. Your brain is adjusting to new ways of functioning. Thinking is fragmented because you are interrupted by baby-related needs. Plus, your brain is also adjusting to keeping track of an exponentially larger task list. You need time and compassion for this adjustment. It won't feel this way forever, and know that your brain is actually fine-tuning itself, becoming more efficient, shedding unnecessary and less important neural networks, and going to be better than ever. We'll continue to talk about ways to help yourself during this process."

Sometimes it's difficult for mothers to understand that their brains are in the process of actually improving their functioning. Therapy during an opportune neuroplastic period is beneficial for treating mental health symptoms and coping with life transitions and stress, and can boost the process of self-discovery and growth.

I believe that my own treatment for postpartum OCD was more successful and brain-changing because I did it at such an integral neurodevelopmental time: in the early months after giving birth. It really changed my relationship with stress to this very day. I rarely think about those stressors now. It seems to me that the neural pathways of healthy thoughts, the ability to stay calm and reason, were solidified because I had maternal brain plasticity in motion and the opportunity to build a better foundation in my brain. Think about it: there is a reason it is easier for young children to learn a new language than adults. It's because children are developing at a much more rapid rate, and neural connections are being developed much more readily. If you are considering therapy, this early phase of parenthood is the time to strike while the iron is hot. Therapy is not just for treating severe symptoms. That is one part of therapy, but I often tell my patients that the deeper work can be done when we are not putting out fires every week. Therapy is your space for you.

I like to tell my patients a story from another patient, whom I treated years ago, which can further illustrate the transformative process. A while back, Holly, a patient who was thinking about becoming pregnant in the near future, confessed that she was worried she would not be a good mother. She told me a story about being on the beach, observing a mother with three young kids: an infant, a toddler, and a young child. It was a particularly windy day, and all of a sudden, a beach umbrella uprooted from the sand and started flying toward them. My patient stated that she did not know what to do. She wasn't frozen, but it took her a little while to understand what was happening. In comparison, she confided that she witnessed that mother with the three littles immediately jump up from her beach chair and grab the umbrella out of the air. Holly internalized this experience as something that was wrong with her, implying that she may not be cut out for motherhood.

I saw it differently. This mother of three young children had her maternal brain fine-tuned and oriented toward caregiving for her children. She was their protector, and because she was still in the very early phase of motherhood, her primary job was to keep her children physically safe. They did not yet have the capacity to protect themselves and were completely dependent on their primary caregiver—their mother. I was not at all surprised to hear that the mother reacted so quickly, seamlessly removing the threat to her children. Her maternal brain was already fine-tuned through the process of having three children, each one upping the level of physical and emotional challenges to which the mother must rise.

The science to support my observation begins in rodent maternal brains. The late Craig Kinsley, PhD, investigated rodent maternal brain plasticity at the University of Richmond. Mother rats, compared to non-mother rats, had improved memory, became less stressed in the face of obstacles, and were better at learning. In his research, he was able to examine the brain activity of maternal rodents and found that more areas of brain are being used in maternal brains during various tasks. While his research focused on rodents, it could be hypothesized that, in the case of what Holly witnessed on the beach, more areas of the mother's brain were activated and greater brain power was at work in helping the mother respond more quickly to the umbrella.

Furthermore, changes to the human maternal brain differ from those in the octopus brain, although the clinician in me can't help but wonder if the octopus's demise is related to perinatal anxiety and depression. I would love to design an experiment with octopus mothers to see if some intense psychotherapy, behavioral activation, and perhaps a boost from psychotropic medication reduces their suicidality.

In human mothers, the peripartum phase and transition to motherhood is the single greatest amount of neurobiological change a mother goes through in the shortest period of time. This developmental phase includes maternal brain, hormonal, and identity changes, and is referred to as matrescence (pronounced similarly to adolescence). During this transition, the brain experiences profound neuroplasticity and parallels the prolific growth that occurs during adolescence. While adolescence can begin as early as 10 years of age, the adolescent brain isn't fully developed into an adult brain until age 26. That's nearly 16 years of a brain adjusting to adolescence and transitioning to adulthood. The transition to motherhood is condensed into a much briefer period, with gestation approximately nine months and then postpartum classified as one year after birth. However, the identity transition to becoming a mother is constant and evolving throughout a lifetime, with a dramatic peak in early motherhood. The physiological hormonal and brain changes are much more pronounced and occur in a much briefer period of time.

SNAPSHOT

The Real Mommy Brain

- The transition to motherhood is called matrescence (pronounced like adolescence).
- During matrescence, the maternal brain experiences profound neuroplasticity and parallels the prolific growth that occurs in adolescence.
- You have little control over these biological changes. Observe how the changes are happening in you. Be open to the process and what it will reveal.
- The maternal brain is reorganizing and fine-tuning itself through processes such as synaptic pruning, increased myelination, grey matter reduction, volume loss, and specialization and refinement of neural networks to prepare your brain for motherhood.

Full disclosure: there is a paucity of maternal brain plasticity research, likely due to male-dominated research programs. It is reported that only 4 percent of research funds are allocated to women's health studies. Much of the available research focuses on fetal development. I encourage the field to increase funding lines and research studies to better understand and support our nation's leading untapped resource: the maternal brain. However, in the past several decades, what research is available yields integral insight to the maternal brain.

THE REAL MOMMY BRAIN • 19

One of the leading researchers on maternal brain plasticity, Else-line Hoekzema, PhD, director of the Hoekzema Lab at the Amsterdam University Medical Center, compared brain scans of pregnant women to nonpregnant counterparts and fathers before and after pregnancy. Her 2017 study revealed significant reductions in grey matter in areas related to social cognition and reductions in areas of the brain that are most responsive to their babies and were predictive of measures of attachment and hostility postpartum. The fMRI scans that revealed changes in grey matter were nonspecific on a neural level. This means that the reductions can indicate any number of physiological changes in neural mechanisms, including dendritic connections, myelination, and number of neurons.

In the same study, Hoekzema and her colleagues found that, on a self-report measure of attachment, grey matter volume reductions were correlated with greater attachment scores and lower hostility toward their babies. What's more, these changes in grey matter remained at the two-year follow-up assessment. The results substantiate that maternal brain changes occur to facilitate the transition to motherhood, rid the brain of unnecessary material, and help it run more efficiently in less space.

The grey matter volume reductions in pregnancy parallel those of adolescence, when the brain is also working to function more efficiently to prepare for adulthood and more developed biopsychosocial functioning. It is also interesting that hippocampal grey matter only increased in the postpartum period (following the pregnancy-related reductions), as the hippocampus is responsible for learning, memory, and encoding. When a mother is born, it is all new learning. The maternal brain gears up to make sure it is in an optimal learning state.

The Real Mommy Brain

* When a mother is born, it is all new learning. Your brain is getting in optimal shape for learning.
* Understanding what you can do to facilitate the transition to motherhood will help you pinpoint how to address your needs and thrive in motherhood.
* Some brain changes last up to two years postdelivery and longer.
* Memory functioning and mommy brain symptoms, such as fogginess, appear to return to near baseline at two years.

In 2022, Pawluski, Hoekzema, and colleagues published a review of the structural and functional maternal brain changes that have been examined to date.[19] Their article highlights the counterintuitive "less is more" phenomenon. The changes are mostly reductions in important characteristics of the maternal brain. When I asked Hoekzema about her latest research, she responded that "in adolescence (a period that is also associated with increases in sex steroid hormones as is the case in pregnancy), there are also strong reductions in grey matter volume. These reductions are thought to represent a specialization and refinement of neural networks. In adolescence, these volume losses are known to at least partially reflect a process of synaptic pruning (i.e., the elimination of weak synapses that renders a more efficient and specialized network)."

Hoekzema further explained, "We don't know yet what the volume reductions in pregnancy represent, and that's impossible to define with certainty when measuring processes in living humans. However, we have found indications that suggest some type of functional specialization takes place in mothers. For instance, we have found that these volume losses predicted stronger mother-infant bonding and a stronger response in brain activation when seeing the infant in the postpartum period. And in current studies (where we have just seen these same changes in brain structure in another independent sample—very exciting), again we are seeing associations with many peripartum maternal processes.[20] So there are indications that these volume losses might at least partially represent an adaptive process that affects the mother's response to her infant.

"It's also interesting that in animal studies some findings point to a process of refinement being associated with the process of triggering maternal care in the mother. However, there is much we don't know yet, and it could also be that what we see represents a mixture of adaptive and degenerative processes, or that some of these adaptations may have less beneficial effects on other processes in the peripartum period."

As my discussion with Hoekzema continued, I drew from my background in clinical psychology and asked her to address the timeline of the postpartum period. In the clinical field, we define the "postpartum" period as up to one year after birth. Based on my work with my patients, I think this is erroneous, as I think postpartum can last longer. I wanted to get some insight into what Hoekzema considered as the postpartum period based on her maternal brain research, which assesses brain changes up to two years postpartum. Hoekzema explained that she doesn't believe there's a very strict cutoff period, and it is likely that you never completely return to your prepregnancy state in terms of your brain. In fact, some brain changes are maintained for two years postpartum. We don't know how long the brain changes last because we simply don't have the studies assessing maternal brain changes long term yet. In one study, Hoekzema reported that the hippocampus, a brain area that is important for memory, was slowly reverting to its prepregnancy state over two years. This aligns with findings showing that memory performance reverts to its prepregnancy state around two years after giving birth. So this suggests that some processes are temporary, while others are maintained for a much longer period. It is reassuring to know that the subjective experience of "fogginess" or negative symptoms associated with mommy brain can get better by two years postpartum.

Pregnancy and becoming a mother are very important transitions that greatly affect your biology and every part of your life. Hoekzema and her colleagues are investigating maternal brain plasticity, including investigating what happens during a second pregnancy, when a woman is exposed to another round of massive hormone surges. Other studies being conceptualized include what happens to other components of the brain, such as brain activity, or environmental changes like sleep loss and stress. More research is needed to understand how these changes affect the mother's behavior, her cognition, and her mental health, as well as how these changes in the mother affect the infant. Hoekzema further explains that knowing more about the maternal brain and motherhood will help us better understand women's brains and the trajectory of changes across the life span. Even mapping these changes in healthy postpartum women represents the first step toward a better understanding of what is happening in women who suffer from perinatal mental health conditions, such as postpartum depression or postpartum psychosis. With every period of heightened neuroplasticity, there is great opportunity and risk. As such, it is a very vulnerable period for the mother, and we should aim to understand the neurobiological processes contributing to more attuned caregiving and serious mental health conditions.

It is no wonder that there are such high rates of postpartum depression and anxiety (PPDA) after childbirth. Many mothers are not aware that their symptoms are postpartum depression and anxiety. How can they be? Their brain is telling them not to pay attention to their own suffering and to focus on the baby. In addition, mothers often do not report their symptoms because they are afraid they will be viewed as "unfit" or not a good mother since depression and anxiety don't align with society's view of the ideal mother.

SNAPSHOT

The Real Mommy Brain

- The peripartum period is a very vulnerable period for both mother and child, particularly for maternal mental health.
- You may experience symptoms of postpartum depression and anxiety up to two years after delivery. It is not your fault. It doesn't mean that you are doing anything wrong. Perinatal depression and anxiety can occur in up to one-third of mothers.
- Motherhood does not happen overnight. It is a process. Be patient and compassionate with yourself. It takes time to settle in to this new role.
- We can use maternal brain plasticity to our advantage to help improve our transition and maternal mental health care.
- When mothers are stressed or struggle, they think they are failing and doing something wrong. But that assumption is flawed.

We have an opportunity to restructure the early parent brain system to our advantage. For example, I mentioned before that there are levels of neurological changes that occur in the transition to motherhood, the hyper (greater brain changes), hypo (lesser brain changes), and typical (average brain changes) responders. What if we knew that you were likely to be a hyper responder? In other words, your brain likely goes into overdrive to attend to baby; you would have to work harder to be more attuned to *your own* needs.

You are probably wondering what about dads? Or other allomothers? Brain changes occur in fathers and other caregivers too. The benefits of child-rearing are not limited to biological mothers as long as the caregivers are actively involved in caregiving. The brain changes occur due to a phenomenon known as phenotypic plasticity—neurological changes among fathers and other non-biological caregivers who are heavily involved in caregiving, resulting from responses to environmental cues from children.[20] Some changes that occur in human fathers include modifications in grey matter and increases in the formation of neural networks and neurons. The greater the involvement, the greater the neuroplastic changes. Ruth Feldman, PhD, Simms-Mann Professor in Developmental Social Neuroscience at the Interdisciplinary Center Herzlia in Israel with a joint appointment at the Yale Child Study Center, stipulates that brain changes in fathers occur from a top-down process, where they cognitively work to anticipate their babies' needs, which changes their brain.

In comparison, mothers are given more of a biological push from deep within their limbic system, and their brain changes occur through a bottom-up approach. Feldman goes on to state that the human paternal brain changes are similar to maternal and other caregiver brain changes and that, taken together, they represent a global human caregiving network. The neural network serves to orient the parental brain to tending to the baby, anticipating and responding to the baby's needs, and thinking beyond the short-term needs of the baby.

In terms of dads and other partners, Milton Kotelchuck, PhD, former professor of pediatrics at Harvard Medical School and principal investigator of the Pregnancy to Early Life Longitudinal database project, has studied the effects of early parenting on paternal mental and physical health. Kotelchuck underscores how monumental the transition to parenthood is for both mothers and fathers. He summarizes the many changes that occur in fathers, even as early as their partner's pregnancy. Testosterone levels decrease while other hormones, such as estradiol, oxytocin, and prolactin, increase. All of this is associated with adaptive bonding and paternal involvement. In addition, these changes parallel the processes that occur in women.

Kotelchuck also goes on to address "dad brain" and the emerging research that highlights more similarities in brain changes between men and women in parenting. While brain plasticity occurs in fathers too, there is one notable sex difference. A father's brain plasticity is stronger in the social-cognitive pathway network.[21] What's important to understand about this specific plasticity change in fathers' brains is that it is related to an increase in mentalizing (e.g., a father's ability to interpret their baby's psychological states). Mothers are able to do this more readily, for both biological and practical reasons of likely spending more time with the infants, so evolution basically gives men's brains a little biological push to get there. Evolutionarily speaking this makes sense because if fathers can anticipate babies' needs and mental states, they can respond more effectively and thus have potentially more positive experiences with their offspring. This is reinforcing and encourages them to be more involved in child-rearing. There are also changes in grey matter, similar to mothers, which further support neuroplastic changes that occur in fathers' brains due to raising babies.

As I have mentioned, we have plasticity on our side, people. While your brain is reorganizing itself to tend to your baby's needs, it's already in motion to tend to "needs." Let's add tending to your own needs as soon as possible and, when applicable, even before the baby's needs. This can mean digging deeper and more creatively into mental health treatment, self-care, and personal enrichment.

For example, when the baby arrives, in the first days in the hospital, accept the help. You are recovering. Allow the nurses to do as much as they can for you and the baby. Start practicing brief intervals of self-care. The first strategy I like to teach my patients is deep breathing or diaphragmatic breathing to relax your mind and body. Try the 4-7-8 breathing technique. Inhale through your nose for four seconds, send the breath down to your belly and get a big Buddha/ pregnant belly, hold the breath in for seven seconds, and exhale out of your mouth for eight seconds. Release all that air and repeat for eight rounds. This takes about two minutes. Practice three to four times a day (bonus if you can do it longer, but most moms do not have a lot of time). The rationale behind inhaling the breath through your nose is that the breath hits the nasal passages and begins to swirl the air as it goes through your body. This is a pleasing sensation to your breathing tubes, and the moistened, swirled air goes to the bottom of the lungs, allowing for a deeper exhale. When you exhale, you release more carbon dioxide out of your system and send more oxygen throughout your blood vessels in your body. This process promotes relaxation.

Use mindfulness to teach your body to relax and reset your nervous system. One brief tactic you can start in the hospital, then continue at home, is to engage in a mindfulness activity while washing your hands. This technique has been studied and tested in research with nurses working in intense hospital units. The same can apply for busy moms. In the hospital, every time you wash your hands (e.g., after going to the bathroom, before you hold your baby), take a deep inhale and focus on the sensations occurring in your hands. What does the water feel like on your skin? What does the running water sound like? What does the soap smell like? Slow down the motions and try to be present washing your hands. These are brief opportunities to reenter your body and get out of your head. During busy shifts, nurses only have the time between taking care of patients to reset. The same can apply to mothers. Remind yourself that washing your hands is a cue to engage your senses. Describe to yourself what you see, hear, smell, and feel. Washing your hands can be a brief but impactful way to calm your nervous system. Continue this practice at home.

When your brain is rewiring to increase anxiety to worry about your baby's needs, your body does not know the difference between "new baby anxiety" and general anxiety. Your body just feels anxious. And you cannot feel physiologically anxious about your baby and relaxed at the same time. It is a global state and all feels the same: anxious. So by relaxing your body, you can reduce anxiety about your baby. When we are relaxed, we are better able to problem-solve, access creativity, learn, and adapt. Know that this is the beginning of learning to nurture your transition to motherhood. In the hospital, focus on small, minute-to-minute, simple strategies. We will get to greater ways to support your maternal development in subsequent chapters.

You can also try lying in that hospital bed doing absolutely nothing but letting your body heal. Or you can shift your thoughts to stretching, or visualizing healing, or watching Bravo, or reading a magazine. It does not have to be profound. It just has to be for *you*. Even if it is only 10 minutes. Even if it is only three minutes. Start there. It's like exercising a muscle when you haven't been to the gym in 10 months. Your hormones are shifting in a new direction to attend to the profound realization that your baby is no longer in your womb and instead is in the real world.

Think of becoming a mother as a sport, and you are the athlete. You want to practice to be in peak performance for tending to your baby. In sports psychology, overthinking and worrying can diminish performance. The same is true in motherhood. Relaxing your body is a way to interrupt the overthinking, new mom worry process that is typical in those early years. It's important to get in the mindset that this is a new "sport" for you; that it's a marathon and not a sprint. You will have to practice (don't worry—you will have endless opportunities), but let's start with developing good form.

When you are ready to think about bigger strategies, keep in mind that exercise, mental stimulation, sleep, diet, and social interaction all nurture neuroplasticity in positive ways. Regular physical exercise has been shown to increase the growth of new brain cells and improve overall brain function. In those early days, moms are not able to exercise while they recover, but even going for a walk and visualizing exercise can have mental health benefits. Engaging in activities that challenge the mind, such as learning a new language or playing brain-training games, can also help to increase plasticity. So go ahead, play Wordledordle or Noodlenerdle or Dordledoodle or another pleasurable brain-exercising game while you are in the hospital or feeding the baby. Plus, an engaging activity can interrupt the new mom worries and anxiety you are likely experiencing. If you're not up for it, don't fret. Parenting will provide plenty of mental stimulation.

Getting enough quality sleep is also important for maintaining overall brain health, including plasticity. While this may seem impossible in the early months, I will discuss strategies for improving sleep in later chapters. Eating a healthy diet that is rich in fruits, vegetables, and omega-3 fatty acids can also support brain health and plasticity. Maintaining social connections and engaging in social activities can help increase plasticity in the brain. Remember: you don't have to do all these things all the time and all at once. They are simply things to be mindful of incorporating where you can.

I know what you are thinking: "Okay, I get it, there are a lot of brain changes in pregnancy and postpartum. All this neurological science, what does it actually mean for me and why should I care? You want me to learn all this on top of everything else I have to do? When should I become a neuroscientist—between feeding and burping and changing the diapers and picking up little Tasha from daycare? Sure, I'll get right on that!"

Slow down a minute. Try to stay with me. Before I tell you what to do with this information, I want to tell you why you should care. I share all this knowledge with you to put you in a place of empowerment. The transition to motherhood is profound. Becoming a mother is its own developmental phase. It is a permanent, one-way ticket, and you will be a different person from the inside out.

The Real Mommy Brain

- Becoming a parent is an opportunity to further develop your brain through experiential plasticity.
- Through parent-child interactions and hormonal and neurological changes, your brain is becoming more efficient and powerful.
- During early motherhood, the parental brain is in prime time for brain plasticity.
- Practice the 4-7-8 diaphragmatic breathing for eight rounds, approximately two minutes, two to three times per day.
- Practice mindfulness techniques, such as washing your hands. What do you see, hear, smell, and feel while you wash your hands? Reenter your body and get out of your head.

3

PREPARE YOUR POSTPARTUM MENTAL HEALTH CARE PLAN

"I wish I knew about postpartum depression. I wish I knew to look out for it. I just thought there was something seriously wrong with me." —HAYDEN PANETTIERE[22]

Now that I have taught you about how the maternal brain works and how to start to nurture its development, I want to talk about some of the very real barriers that get in the way of your maternal brain development and how to prepare for them and remove them. If you had asked me to describe myself pre-baby, I would say that I was no stranger to struggling. In fact, by the time I had reached my thirties, I considered myself a professional coper with anxiety. Having always been a worrier, I have spent years refining my coping strategies through therapy, exercise, socializing, and self-care. I am a seasoned patient in psychotherapy, and there is nothing about myself that I am not willing to explore. Before becoming a mother, I believed that I had simply done the work.

If once before every menstrual cycle I had the thought that I would die of a particular type of cancer, it would not alarm me. I had become accustomed to a certain baseline level of health anxiety. In response,

I would go for a run, meet a friend for a drink, or talk about it with my therapist. As a result, I could reliably assume that any outlandish thought would go away with a reasonable amount of problem-solving.

My professional role allows me to move through my own internal obstacles to help my patients. If you only know me in my professional role, you may never know that I am prone to worry at times of stress. I can easily distract myself with other people's worries, and I'm particularly drawn to help other patients with anxiety. The neurotic mind does not scare me. In fact, the more eccentric the worry, the more connected I feel.

Prior to motherhood, I designed my life to be able to cope with whatever was thrown at me. My strategies were refined, perfected, intact, and ready to be implemented at a moment's notice. I was self-aware, brave, curious, and accustomed to being analytical. I figured that I would sail through the rest of my life, given that I was so good at taking care of myself. I entered into motherhood with a certain hubris that I could not be more prepared for this transition. However, the joke was on me. And it wasn't funny.

About a year after my husband and I got married, our daughter, Jordan, was born. Due to early challenges with breastfeeding, I pumped and bottle-fed. The breastfeeding challenges early on were not something I could have predicted. I had always planned to breastfeed and just assumed it would happen easily. Jordan was born four weeks early and had jaundice. This made her lethargic, and while she could latch and feed, she had trouble staying awake while feeding. In addition, it took a while to wake her up every hour and get her into the feeding. I was anxious that she was not getting enough to eat. She also needed the breastmilk to help her recover from jaundice. It felt like I was always up against the clock. I began pumping so I could keep track of her intake and so that she could feed more quickly. The once 30-minute routine was now a 90-minute extravaganza to pump, bottle-feed, burp, diaper change, and get Jordan back to sleep. Never mind wash, dry, and prepare pump parts and bottles for the next shift. This left me with, best case scenario, a two-hour sleeping window between feedings *if* I could fall back asleep quickly, which was almost never the case.

The lack of sleep after Jordan was born was torture. I knew that deficits in sleep would impact my mood in a negative way, as it does for so many. It began taking its toll. I reached out to my psychotherapist, Dr. Nancy, for support while my sleep was dwindling. With the added support and guidance on how to navigate these unforeseen challenges, over time I was able to keep up with breastfeeding. When I was ready, and about eight months into postpartum, I started to wean from pumping and intermittently breastfeeding. While I knew to wean gradually, the hormonal shift was so intense and my anxiety ramped up so much that I suffered from postpartum OCD. Dr. Nancy explained this to me, and it was as if I had not been specializing in treating patients with OCD for years. I always knew that I had anxiety, but postpartum OCD? She explained that my avoidance and preoccupation with protecting Jordan was more than being a new mom. I thought, what's wrong with avoiding public bathrooms and mommy-and-me classes, or not letting friends over if they had other children in daycare (aka the petri dish), or questioning relatives about their other social engagements and cold symptoms? So you're telling me it's not okay to mentally calculate visitors' exposure to germs plus incubation time to potential period of contagion? Let me remind you, this was all way before COVID existed. Isn't this just being careful with a new baby?

"It is," she said, "but not when it is a constant preoccupation and causing you distress. Plus, you are checking." Checking, in anxiety, means that you seek an answer for the uncertainty. An example of checking is wondering, "Is this new rash cancerous?" and then looking at online images of cancerous rashes and comparing them to the spots on your baby's skin. If the spot looks nothing like the images, relief is experienced.

In the research, it turns out that postpartum mothers are more likely to develop OCD. The base rate in the general population for OCD is 1 to 2 percent. However, in postpartum mothers, the prevalence rate increases to 9 percent.[23] This makes sense because the postpartum brain is becoming more attuned and vigilant to take care of the baby. Anxiety naturally increases when you have a baby.

Postpartum depression is also common and can co-occur with anxiety and OCD. Some common symptoms of depression include trouble sleeping, loss of interest, excessive guilt, loss of energy, difficulty concentrating (some of this is typical in early motherhood), changes in appetite, moving more slowly than usual (and not due to medical recovery from birth, C-section, or pain), and suicidal thoughts. It is important if you are feeling off to let a medical professional assess your symptoms. You do not need to diagnose yourself. Also, because early motherhood brings with it normative sleep challenges and changes in attention, it is important to let a doctor more thoroughly assess your mood, taking all these factors into account.

> "You have so many new jobs as a mother. Let the doctors do theirs."

Postpartum OCD is different from the common intrusive thoughts that are experienced by up to 90 percent of new parents. Thoughts such as "What if I harm the baby?" or "What if I accidentally drop the baby?" are intrusive thoughts. These are harmless and also very typical in early parenthood. These thoughts are anxious thoughts. Anxiety and OCD are different mental health conditions. The most current research defines OCD as a dysfunction of executive functioning, while anxiety is considered to be rooted in emotional processing.

Intrusive thoughts can also be characteristic of postpartum OCD when parents are preoccupied by the thoughts, avoid things because they think the thoughts are true, or experience a high level of distress from the thoughts. They can also be part of normal adjustment to parenthood. In Karen Klieman's book, *Good Moms Have Scary Thoughts*, she offers validation for intrusive thoughts that many mothers and fathers experience in early parenthood. However, when worries become preoccupations or obsessions, lead to avoidance, and cause a level of distress that interferes with functioning or ability to enjoy daily life, then a clinical disorder may be present and may benefit from treatment. There is no cure for OCD or postpartum OCD; however, with treatment, we can turn down the volume greatly and help mothers get the relief they need.

In my practice, my personal experience and professional training have given me a nuanced ear to diagnose postpartum OCD. It is often that it has been missed or patients are misdiagnosed because their seemingly "normal mom worries" sound reasonable. But, with further assessment, it becomes clear that the worries interfere with their ability to experience pleasure in this phase in motherhood. There is also a culture of martyrdom around motherhood, where a certain level of suffering is "just part of being a new mom." I disagree. A lot of mothers are suffering more than they need to, even in this phase of real challenges. When I hear my patients say, "I can't sleep at night. I check to see if the baby is breathing and have to keep the baby monitor on my pillow," I probe further. "I am delaying giving my baby solid foods because I am so scared they will choke," I inquire more. "I can't let anyone hold the baby because I am afraid they will get her sick" and "I won't take my baby out in public because I am afraid I will forget to take my baby out of the car" require more assessment.

To give you another example, I came to terms with my diagnosis of postpartum OCD as not just the more common experiences of intrusive thoughts when I called Poison Control. Because it was flu season, I had plenty of hand sanitizer strategically placed throughout our home. I even had a bottle on Jordan's changing table. One time, I pumped the bottle too hard and sanitizer flew across the table. I became terrified because I didn't see where the sanitizer landed. Did it land in Jordan's mouth as she lay there on her back? Her mouth is open!! I didn't see it go into her mouth, but how could I be sure? I Googled it immediately.

"Children can be at risk for alcohol poisoning if any more than *a taste* of hand sanitizer is ingested. . . . Symptoms include confusion, vomiting, respiratory arrest, and death." What exactly constituted a "taste" of hand sanitizer? Was that less than one pump? You may be saying to yourself, "Well, that's ridiculous. A taste is clearly the amount in question." If you are thinking that, congratulations, you've never had postpartum OCD. Or maybe you did and got treatment and now recognize that this is an absurd line of thinking, as I do now. But when you have postpartum OCD, as I did, you take your nose and stick it completely in your baby's mouth and start sniffing. When you don't smell anything and are still unsure, you call Poison Control. The man on the other end of the phone is nice and reassuring, and you realize this is the same guy who answered last week when you mistakenly thought Jordan drank baby shampoo. Don't they rotate responders?! Embarrassed, you hang up and call your physician husband and cry that you may or may not have accidentally poisoned your baby. You tell your psychotherapist what happened, and you increase your therapy sessions to twice weekly.

Dr. Nancy and I spent the next several months tackling the postpartum OCD together and adjusting to new motherhood. During this time, it did not help that I also developed a mysterious skin condition. I came home from the gym one day and noticed that my arms were covered in red splotches. I thought I had an allergic reaction to my post-workout smoothie, took a Benadryl, and thought little of it. But the splotches kept appearing all over my body. They would occur after I did the things I usually enjoy, such as drinking a glass of red wine, rigorous exercise, being outside in the sun, and taking hot showers and baths. The first doctor I saw ran a bunch of tests and ruled out anything serious. He told me that I had heat-induced cholinergic urticaria. Basically, I had become allergic to my body temperature changing from heat. The kicker? He said that the bodily response can *sometimes* trigger anaphylaxis. As I listened to him speak, I tried to make sense of how my body was now allergic to my favorite pastimes. That anytime

I tried to enjoy myself, I could potentially have a life-threatening reaction. This is the last thing a mother wants to hear. Now I would have to play Russian roulette with my self-care and pleasurable activities?! I realized I needed treatment for this anxiety too.

Some of the most effective treatments for mental illness are counterintuitive. The intuitive response to anxiety is to avoid what makes you anxious. For example, evolutionarily speaking, the caveman sees a tiger in the wild and runs away. However, the best treatment for anxiety is cognitive behavioral therapy plus exposure. For OCD and postpartum OCD, it is a specific treatment called cognitive behavioral therapy plus exposure and response prevention. The treatment requires you to engage in activities that will increase your anxiety; it teaches you to face your fears. This is not how we have adapted in evolution. We would have never survived if our caveman brain told us that when we see a tiger in the wild, *run after the tiger*. No one wants to run after the tiger, yet that is the treatment.

In treatment with Dr. Nancy, we just added the hive-inducing activities to the already exponentially growing list of exposures for postpartum OCD. My exposures for postpartum OCD included saying yes to all baby activity plans (yes, even indoor play gym birthday parties), not asking visitors questions about illness symptoms or exposure to viruses (again, all before COVID existed), making myself use public bathrooms and changing tables to change Jordan's diaper, and allowing her to play with the shared toys at the pediatrician's office.

For treatment for anxiety about hives, with my EpiPen in tow, I ran on a hot day, did a spin class, took a shower, took Jordan to play on the beach in July humidity, and ordered red wine when I went out to dinner. I know what you are thinking—that all sounds pretty good for the most part. It sure used to be, before I learned that I could spontaneously die at any moment. Once I was exposed to the heat, the rash would cover my body and I would wait in terror for the anaphylaxis that would or would not develop for at least 30 minutes because "it's a delayed reaction, not immediate," my doctor said. The onset of death would commence, or the rash would simply go away and nothing would happen. This seemed like a cruel joke for a new mom to have to endure with all the other challenges that happen in those early months with a baby.

A lot of new moms with anxiety are scared to be home alone with their babies when they have anxiety. I happened to be afraid of being home alone with Jordan in case I had an anaphylactic reaction and died and left her without a mother. In the height of my anxiety, I would even wait until Mike got home to take a shower, or I would avoid going for long walks on really hot days when it was just me and Jordan. With treatment, I got better. I tell you this because, with treatment, even though I still have cholinergic urticaria, I forget I have it. Most of the time I don't even notice the hives. It doesn't even cross my mind anymore that I could have an anaphylactic reaction after a workout. This is what good treatment can do for postpartum OCD. Or, as Dr. Nancy liked to frame it, "The problem is not the urticaria. The problem is the anxiety."

As new mothers, we are biologically primed to be anxious, to pro-tect our completely dependent babies. That's a lot of pressure. Often, we can become hyperfocused on the situation at hand, the specific thing that is "scary," when really we need to take a step back, treat the anxiety underneath, and use our strategies to manage triggers. More often than not, it's not an emergency, even when it feels like one. In early motherhood, we forget that we have never done this before, or even if we have, now it's different.

The point of OCD and anxiety treatment is to desensitize you enough and allow you to learn new coping so that the event is not triggering. It does not mean that there is no risk of something bad happening. A current marker of treatment success is that I don't even think twice when Jordan has to go number two in the bathrooms at restaurants—her new favorite pastime! She insists we go several times at each meal. Another marker of success occurred last week, when Jordan sneezed into my eyeball while she was sick with the flu. Without a flinch, I responded, "Wow, you are making my immune system so strong," and then I forgot about it.

For mothers who feel "off" and are suffering in any way, I always recommend they seek advice from a licensed mental health provider or member of their medical team. The current standard of care is to have a postpartum mental health visit within the first six weeks after birth. However, that is not always followed. When I was researching this topic, I spoke to several OB-GYNs to see what they did in their practices. The results were mixed. Dr. Jessica Vernon, the former obstetric director of perinatal mental health at NYU Langone and current associate medical director and clinical director of product development at Oula, does a two-week check-in. If she has a high-risk patient, she will monitor them more frequently. She explains that she often has to create a warm, trusting environment quickly so that mothers can feel safe reporting symptoms. We both agreed that the earlier, the better. I often recommend mothers establish care with a psychiatrist and psychologist or other certified postpartum mental health professional early on in pregnancy or before becoming pregnant. In addition, schedule follow-up visits and have frequent check-ins with your providers. Providers should be on alert when you deliver, during the weeks after, and at regular intervals given that postpartum conditions can occur any time during the first year or later. Build your support team early so that providers can get a good baseline assessment of your mood and history, and so that they are not first meeting you in crisis. Channeling my best Oprah voice, I say to mothers, "You get a therapist, and you get a therapist, you all get a therapist!"

For milder cases of perinatal depression and anxiety, supportive and talk therapy can be enough. You may or may not be familiar with the research that indicates that the therapeutic relationship is the most important factor in effective therapy. That is only the case when the symptoms are mild. If you have more severe symptoms, treatment modality matters. In other words, it is important to find a provider who is skilled at treating postpartum mental illness and using evidence-based therapies, such as cognitive behavioral therapy with exposure for anxiety, behavioral activation for depression, and exposure and response prevention for OCD.

When symptoms are more severe, medication can be instrumental. Recently, the Food and Drug Administration approved the first drug specifically for treating postpartum depression. The medication is meant to be short acting, and the course of treatment is two weeks. In clinical trials, symptom relief was achieved in as little as three days. This is incredible progress in treating postpartum depression. Just a caveat: medications used to treat depression will still work for postpartum depression; however, these medications can often take weeks to take effect. So this is great news because another medication option for treating postpartum depression that is quick and effective will save more lives.

It can also be helpful to strategically schedule your postpartum mental health visits around common contributors to perinatal mood disorders. For example, if you are having trouble sleeping for many consecutive days, or feel unable to get any pleasure, or have begun weaning from breastfeeding, it may be time to check in with your provider. We tend to see two spikes in postpartum mood disorders based on the hormonal shifts of breastfeeding. Right after birth is common when the mother is not breastfeeding. This does not include baby blues, which last two to three days and not longer than one week. The second common timepoint of postpartum occurrence is at the time of weaning or stopping breastfeeding. So it can be very helpful to the mother to schedule mental health visits that align with these shifts.

Prepare Your Postpartum Mental Health Care Plan

- Establish your postpartum mental health care team *before* you have your baby.
- Cognitive Behavioral Therapy is very effective for symptoms of depression, anxiety, and OCD. Treatment can be counterintuitive: face your fears for anxiety, resist compulsions for OCD, and make yourself do activities for depression.
- Up to 90 percent of new parents have intrusive thoughts (e.g., thoughts about harm to the baby).
- Contact and meet with a psychotherapist (or several) in the months prior to childbirth to decide who you want to work with if you want or need therapy postpartum. It may take several tries with different clinicians to figure out which therapist works best for you.
- Once you pick a therapist, schedule your first follow-up appointment at two weeks postdelivery.

Sleep is one of the most important mood stabilizers. Lack of sleep can trigger a host of mental health conditions, including increased postpartum anxiety, depression, episodes of mania, and psychosis. The current recommendation for postpartum care stipulates that you do whatever it takes to let new mothers sleep. Sleep is incredibly restorative and protective for mental health. When so many factors are against you, make sleep a priority. Work with your partner and support system to figure out how you can protect your sleep at all costs. There are many ways to protect a good stretch (five to six hours of sleep) in the evening. It is more restorative if mothers get their longest stretch in the earlier part of the evening, with more hours before midnight. However, if you are used to being a night owl, then after midnight may be more helpful for you. Consider your own preferences.

Have the sleep schedule set one month before your due date. Psychologically prepare yourself and your partner to adhere to the schedule for at least three months. It is helpful to discuss this sleep schedule timeline with your partner so that you both can set realistic expectations. Depending on your unique situation, the sleep schedule may need to be upheld longer than three months; alternatively, it may not be needed that long. Either way, you are more prepared.

Consider supplementing with formula or pumping so that someone else—a partner, a relative, baby nurse, nanny, babysitter, friend—can take over one feeding. Use a calendar to map out coverage and a rotation of help if needed. If nothing else, sleep for the mother (primary caregiver), should be a top priority due to hormonal changes, interrupted sleep at other times, and the stress of filling a new role.

I teach my patients good sleep hygiene strategies to help them improve their sleep quality. As best you can, try to have a regular sleep and wake time. Of course, this is especially challenging in those early months of taking care of a baby. This is why it can be especially helpful to map out a sleeping schedule with a partner and

> Remember: "Do whatever you can to allow new mothers to sleep."

to adhere to it. Also, the bed should only be used for sleep (and sex—I know that's not even on the table right now and may not be for quite some time). This way, when your body gets into bed, it is associated with sleep. Try not to watch television or use your phones in bed. This is because these actions can be activating, making it more difficult than it already is to fall asleep with a newborn. You do not want your body to associate the bed with wakefulness because then it gets confused when it is time to sleep. If you have a comfortable sofa or chair, sit there to do feedings, pumping, scrolling, and any other wakeful activities. I know it's easier said than done. These are not hard-and-fast rules; they are sleep hygiene strategies that can help even when the newborn phase is working against you. Other tactics include making sure your bedroom temperature is set to 68 degrees or a comfortable temperature. If the room is too hot or too cold, it will be difficult to sleep. Also, try to make sure the room is dark.

Prepare Your Postpartum Mental Health Care Plan

- Early motherhood can be an optimal time to start therapy because the maternal brain is primed for learning.
- If you choose to breastfeed, schedule mental health appointments at the time of weaning. At a minimum, you should schedule at least three postpartum mental health visits with a therapist.
- Establish care with a psychiatrist for consultation about medication before you have your baby, even if you do not think you will need it. This way, you can have your care team ready to provide care, and you won't have to scramble last minute to find a provider or get an appointment. You don't want one more thing to do after the baby comes. By setting up the village ahead of time, all you have to do is show up to your appointments.
- Medication and therapy work synergistically, especially in the beginning of therapy. When symptoms are so severe that you cannot do the therapy, medication can help give you that kick start.
- Let the doctors do their jobs and assess you for symptoms of anxiety and depression. You do not have to figure it out on your own.
- Create a protected sleep calendar and schedule protected sleep (at least five to six hours) for the primary caregiver/mother. Enlist others for help—partner, relatives, friends, hired help—and create and adhere to a rotation.
- Try to apply some sleep hygiene strategies when you can.

In addition to postpartum anxiety and depression, a new baseline level of normal new mom worries is established after you have a baby. Despite the influx of new things to worry about, there are many things you can do to manage new mom worries and anxiety. I will go in depth about this more in a later chapter, but here are a few general strategies to keep in mind. There are two categories of coping strategies: emotion-focused and problem-solving coping. First, ask yourself, "Is this in my control or not?" If the worry is in your control (e.g., what if my baby is not eating enough?), then problem-solve. Meet with a pediatrician to assess weight gain, bottle-feed, weigh baby before and after feedings, and assess output. If the worry is not in your control (e.g., what if my baby gets sick?), then it is best to rely on emotion-focused coping strategies. Emotion-focused coping strategies are used to get your mind off the worry because there is no point in thinking about something that is out of your control and, by focusing on it, you will only feel worse.

My favorite emotion-focused coping strategies that I recommend to my patients and will explain further include distraction, deep breathing relaxation, mindfulness, face blanching, and circling every other *a*. I also focus on shorter strategies because I know mom time is limited. Distraction can include calling a friend to get your mind off the worry (not to discuss the worry), exercising, going for a walk outside, listening to a podcast, reading a book, or listening to music. Deep breathing that I went over in chapter 2 is also integral for emotion-focused coping. Remember the 4-7-8 breath and repeat it eight times; practice two to four times a day for two minutes each. Then relax into gentle breathing.

For mindfulness, try the 5-4-3-2-1 method. Take a deep breath, settle into your body, and name five things you can see around you. Then name four things you can touch; if you want, touch them and notice what they feel like. Name three things you can hear; close your eyes to isolate your hearing sense more. Then name two things you can smell. Finally, name one thing you can taste. Another mindfulness exercise I like to recommend is to listen for the most distant sound you can hear. For this, settle into a chair, take three full-belly breaths, and close your eyes. Then listen for the farthest sound you can hear. For example, you may hear the hum of an air conditioner or heater, or traffic outside, or a bird call or voices in a hallway. There are lots of other mindfulness exercises out there; these are just two examples to get you going.

With new mom worries and anxiety, it's important to slow things down. Another strategy is to schedule "mommy worry time." It's like mommy wine time but way less fun and way more necessary for anxiety. Set a timer and allow yourself to worry, cry, imagine worst-case scenarios, but for 10 minutes only, no more than once per day. When the timer goes off, that's it. Follow up worry time with a pleasurable or distracting activity. Say to yourself, "I am not going to think about this now. I am going to allow myself to think about this at my next mommy worry time." Then make a brief note in your phone to refer back to at your next worry time.

The use of personal mantras early on can be very helpful as you are adjusting to new motherhood. I will go into more detail about the cognitive strategies in later chapters. But for now here are two that can help calm the mind. When you don't want to change another diaper, get out of bed in the middle of the night, soothe a fussy baby, or complete other difficult tasks, try thinking, *I don't want to and I will.* This validates your feeling of not wanting to and also honors your commitment to do the thing anyway. Choosing to do even if you don't want to is a hallmark of being a parent. I wish it were easier—it isn't.

Another mantra that is particularly useful in motherhood is "It doesn't have to be perfect to be okay." Repeat this to yourself when you have trouble folding the perfect swaddle or you're not feeling your best moodwise. You can also say it when the house is a mess, there's laundry piling up, you don't have the perfect coordinated outfit for the baby's outings, or the pictures of you postpartum look nothing like that momfluencer on social media. Any pictures you see on social media that don't have a mom looking overwhelmed, surrounded by mess, and with clothes full of spit-up are lies anyway. LIES, I tell you.

I recommend my patients create a mommy coping card with a list of these strategies to refer to. So I did that for you. Here is a Snapshot of a coping card for you. Of course, feel free to make your own and update the list of strategies as you learn new methods that work for you.

SNAPSHOT

Prepare Your Postpartum Mental Health Care Plan

- Be present and engage in mindfulness activities.
- Mindfulness Activity 1: Try the 5-4-3-2-1 exercise. Take a couple deep breaths and notice five things you can see, four things you can touch, three things you can hear, two things you can smell, and one thing you can taste.
- Mindfulness Activity 2: Close your eyes, settle into your chair, take some deep breaths, and listen for the most distant sound you can hear in the background.
- When you have intrusive thoughts or worries, grab a book, newspaper, or magazine, then go line by line and circle every other *a*. It is really difficult to pay attention to intrusive thoughts while you are concentrating on this task.
- Fill a bowl with ice water and stick your face in it to combat intrusive thoughts and worries. Doing this resets your arousal system.
- Use your mommy mantras: "I don't want to and I will" and "It doesn't have to be perfect to be okay."

It is also helpful to prepare a father's postpartum mental health care plan, given that the rate of postpartum depression in fathers is about 10 percent. When I spoke with Dr. Kotelchuck, we discussed the parallel processes that occur for both mothers and fathers, not only in neurological changes but also in the need for improving access to mental health care and more research to understand the nuances of the adaptive changes that happen in paternal brains to ensure parenting capabilities. Kotelchuck confirmed that the brain is really plastic. He astutely noted that perinatal appointments are integral touch points where fathers can be assessed for postpartum depression and anxiety because "the fathers are just in the waiting rooms and no one is talking to them." In fact, his team conducted his research studies with fathers by approaching them in the waiting room.

Kotelchuck and I agreed that perinatal appointments are an opportune time to empower and educate fathers (in addition to mothers) about this profound developmental stage and the changes that will occur during early parenthood. This can include acknowledging the enormity of the transition to parenthood and risk for postpartum depression and anxiety, as well as validating intrusive thoughts. It is also a chance to provide psychoeducation about neurological changes, the health benefits of being more involved in child-rearing, and what to look out for in terms of signs and symptoms of postpartum depression and anxiety in their partners and themselves. Kotelchuck further stated that "it's an opportunity to encourage fathers to be even more involved, and the earlier they get involved, the better, as their biology and sensitivity can aid this process in the early phase of child-rearing."

For mothers, fathers, and other primary caregivers, support groups can be helpful. I recommend looking at the Postpartum Support International website for their available groups. They have a support group for everything. They have support coordinators in every state and over 40 countries. Their support groups range from miscarriages, to postpartum, to paternal depression, to LGBTQ groups and more. Support groups can help with social support in addition to therapeutic treatments. Virtual groups are a convenient option, and you will likely be able to get in immediately, which can bridge the gap until your next mental health appointment.

These are the minimum recommended maternal mental health appointments. Give a copy of this form to your partner to remind you of your appointments and so they have contact information for your medical team.

POSTPARTUM MENTAL HEALTH PLAN

My Name: _____ DOB:_____

My Due Date: _____

Scheduled Delivery / C-Section?   Yes / No

My OB Provider: _____

Hospital Name: _____

My Feeding Plan: Breastfeed / Formula/ Not Sure (circle) and describe:

_____

My mental health therapist who has agreed to follow up with me after delivery:

Therapist Name: _____ Phone Number: _____

Address of Provider: _____

Follow-Up Appointment Days/Times:

APPOINTMENT 1

(intake / baseline assessment at least one month before giving birth)

Date: _____ Time:_____

Location: Virtual telehealth / In-person (circle)

APPOINTMENT 2

(recommended at three weeks post delivery)

Date: _____ Time:_____

Location: Virtual telehealth / In-person (circle)

APPOINTMENT 3

(provider-recommended date or two weeks after starting weaning / stopping breastfeeding)

Date:_____ Time:_____

Location: Virtual telehealth / In-person (circle)

My psychiatrist or prescribing doctor who has agreed to follow up with me after delivery:

Prescriber Name: _____ Phone Number: _____

Address of Provider: _____

Follow-Up Appointment Days/Times:

APPOINTMENT 1

(intake / baseline assessment at least one month before giving birth)

Date: _____ Time:_____

Location: Virtual telehealth / In-person (circle)

APPOINTMENT 2

(recommended within one month of giving birth)

Date: _____ Time:_____

Location: Virtual telehealth / In-person (circle)

APPOINTMENT 3

(recommended two weeks after starting weaning or stopping breastfeeding)

Date: _____ Time:_____

Location: Virtual telehealth / In-person (circle)

4

MATRESCENCE AND THE TRANSITION TO MOTHERHOOD

"I was one of them now, the mothers."
—ASHLEY AUDRAIN, *THE PUSH*

Matrescence, a term coined by medical anthropologist Dana Raphael in 1973, refers to the transition to motherhood and includes the physiological, emotional, and hormonal changes that occur. Mothers also need to understand that while the biological transformation to motherhood is speedy, the psychological transition to motherhood is a gradual process. In graduate school, I was fortunate enough to study behavior change from the founder of the transtheoretical model himself, the late James Prochaska, PhD. That's like taking a psychology course on psychoanalytic case conceptualization from Sigmund Freud. On the first day of class, we were handed a binder of 55 scientific articles to familiarize ourselves with the tenets of the transtheoretical model of behavior change. I was so excited to be learning from one of the greats that I read every single article front to back, integrated that knowledge, and by the end of my graduate training, understood the principles of behavior change inside and out.

Most importantly, and a phenomenon that I discuss often with my patients, is the process of change. Behavior change is never linear. Becoming a mother is a one-way ticket, but it is not a direct linear process. A lot of moms expect that they should just keep moving forward with no hiccups, mistakes, or failures. Therefore, when the process hits a challenge that sets them back, they think the flaw is within them. I work with innumerable mothers to normalize the process of becoming a mother and the progression of success. As you will learn, one of the rules of development is that with every progression there is regression. Motherhood is a developmental phase. As you move forward (progression) through the developmental process, there will be setbacks (regressions) that make you feel that you have failed and are a beginner again. Picture an upward spiral of behavior change. Keep in mind that you never move backward; you just move further up the spiral and hit similar setbacks and challenges. But you approach each setback with more experience, knowledge, practice, and coping strategies, and thus keep moving forward.

---SNAPSHOT---

Matrescence and the Transition to Motherhood

- Matrescence, the process of becoming a mother, is gradual, occurs over time, and is not linear.
- Think of an upward spiral to represent the transition to motherhood: you are moving forward each time but hitting regressions along the way.
- You are always moving forward in the spiral because you come to each regression with more experience, more knowledge, and more ways to cope.

Remember, there is no evolutionary or biological advantage to focusing on ourselves while becoming a mother. You will be pulled to attend to the baby. However, it is psychologically beneficial to nurture yourself through this process. In modern-day motherhood, we can do better because we have fewer environmental threats to keep the baby alive. Ultimately, a mother who is tending to her own needs and her baby's needs is optimal, but you will have to work against biological drives to do so.

What else fades as we become mothers? Certainly, a sense of an independent self. A *New York Times* article described a woman who spoke about her transition to motherhood and the ambivalence she experienced.[24] Not ambivalent in a sense of not caring one way or another, but really caring a great deal in two opposing directions. The writer rightly advocated to normalize contradictory feelings in motherhood, and I could not agree more.

Before baby, it is simply me. Now it is baby and me. *And* is my favorite word in therapy. It is a great rule in improvisational comedy; with it, the scene moves forward into interesting places. Without it, the scene dies. It's an opportunity to lean more in to yes. Of course, it's much easier to lean in to yes when you have slept well, eaten well, are not "touched out," and are not riddled by anxiety and depression.

As I've explained, those three simple letters bridge the most complicated human processes together—the ability to hold opposing feelings at the same time, which is the essence of motherhood. It's very complicated to biologically and lovingly be driven to take care of your baby and to have self-interests pulling you away from baby. However, those three little letters are space, a pause, and consideration. The word *and* is the most hopeful word in the English dictionary. More mothers need to focus on the *and*.

In matrescence, mastering the usage of *and* is essential. *And* is the acceptance of the complexities in motherhood. *And* is tolerance, patience, and love for yourself. I love my babies, and I want them to go to bed immediately. I feel like my heart will explode out of my chest because I love them so much, and I need to get out of the house. I want to spend time with my babies, and I want to work on my career. I am a good mother, and I have bad thoughts about my little ones. I love being a mother, and I want to not have the responsibilities of being a mother. I enjoy my life with my babies, and I miss my life pre-baby. I am bored with the monotony of infancy, and my favorite moments are to be doing nothing else but giggling and smiling with my baby. I want them to grow out of this incredibly hard developmental stage, and I miss the baby phase. I am a good mother, and I don't enjoy every moment. I have sacrificed so much as a mother, and I have gained so much. I made mistakes in mothering today, and I had a great day. I need to take care of my baby, and I need to take care of myself first.

In therapy, *and* represents the dialectic and is described by Marsha Linehan, a psychologist and founder of dialectical behavioral therapy, as the middle ground between two opposing ways of thinking. There is no more powerful word in therapy than the word *and*. Consider a very depressed patient who says, "I don't want to live anymore." You sit, you discuss, and you reflect, "You don't want to live anymore, and yet you have made the choice to come here and fight to live." Or a very anxious patient who is afraid of driving on the highway after getting in a traumatic car accident. The patient says, "I am so afraid of driving on the highway. I can't do it." The most effective therapy works when a patient can hold fear and do the exposures simultaneously, accepting their experience. Exposures are the ultimate form of *and*. *I am terrified of driving on the highway, and I am going to try it again.*

SNAPSHOT

Matrescence and the Transition to Motherhood

- We need to normalize the realities and complexities in motherhood, and promote honesty.
- In development, with every progression, there is regression.
- Let go of what you expected to do as a mother.
- Let go of what everyone else expected you to do as a mother.
- Becoming a mother is a process. Allow the process to unfold to discover the mother who you actually *want* to be. This is on-the-job training and discovery.
- Embrace using "and" statements in motherhood to hold two truths together.

When I first became a mother, I did not expect longing to develop as a mother. My soul yearned for answers to deeper questions: How will I mother my babies? What do I want to imprint on them when they experience me? How can I access a deep nurturing place when there are so many distractions to prevent me from digging deeper into mothering—when the baby needs daycare drop-offs and mommy-and-me activities, and tummy time and stimulation, and solids and purées, and baths and clean laundry? Every time I tried to adhere strictly to "parenting" advice, such as regimented naps or some version of cry it out for sleep training, I became a worse mother. The rules, the "shoulds" and "shouldn'ts," the template for how to get the result I wanted through rigid steps ultimately became more important than what was happening in the room. I began missing the forest for the trees.

How can I access that version of the mother I want to be when there are so many needs pulling at me and none of them are my own?

Mothering is defined as relating to or characteristic of a mother, especially in being caring, protective, and kind. Parenting is the archi-tecture of decisions, discipline, and strategies we put in place when raising our children. In the words of Annie Duke, former professional poker player and author in cognitive-behavioral decision science and education, "The currency of poker is good decisions, not money won." I would argue that the currency of mothering is good decisions, not outcomes. As a society of mothers, we have evolved to do less mothering to ourselves. To mother, in other words, means a shift toward the primacy of what mothers *need* to thrive and a shift away from what children *want* in the moment they're in (and there's a guarantee that comes with each child that she wants something at every moment).

Pilyoung Kim, PhD, associate professor at the University of Denver, researches parenting during the early postpartum months, a stressful and demanding time. One study by Kim and colleagues investigated mothers in poverty who were exposed to higher levels of stress, violence, and noise. Their study found increased amygdala activation in mothers' brains. The amygdala is responsible for detecting threats and rewarding cues. Mothers who were not living in poverty experienced increased amygdala activation to their babies smiling, while mothers living in poverty experienced increased activation in response to their babies crying. This increased activation led to greater intrusiveness for anxious mothers in that they would direct their babies to play in certain ways and play with certain toys. In other words, non-anxious mothers were more open to following infant cues and more flexible in allowing their babies to freely play. Kim expanded, saying that the increased environmental threats lead to more pressure on mothers and fewer moments to relax. To me, this research further reinforces that the less stressed and anxious mothers feel, the less they need to control in parenting. Remember, try to do less parenting and more mothering. If we can tend to our own emotions and mother ourselves, we will be able to tolerate our child's emotions better, allowing them more time to sort it out or cope with their distress.

In challenging moments with your child, take a step back and ask yourself what you need in this moment. I guarantee that if you can figure out how to give yourself what you need, the situation with your child will resolve more fluidly. For example, if your baby is inconsolable, parenting would take a limited approach and ask, "How do I respond to the child?" Instead, a counterintuitive, mother-centric approach would be to ask, "How am I feeling in this moment? Am I feeling powerless, scared, or angry? If so, how can I tend to these feelings *so that I am better able to problem-solve and help soothe my baby?*"

Perhaps it means taking deep breaths and doing something in the moment that makes you feel powerful to counteract the feeling of powerlessness. You could remind yourself of something you did that day that was powerful, or send off that assertive email later, or do a warrior yoga pose, or even take a moment to silently scream at your baby for keeping you up all night in your head. Don't worry, the baby can't read your mind.

Satisfy your need and get to a better mental place, which will allow you to respond more flexibly. A crying baby needs a caregiver who is regulated and grounded. By resolving the emotion that is keeping you caught up in your head, you are mothering yourself. By tending to your needs first, you bring a clearer version of the mother you want to be to the situation. You may find yourself more able to access humor, softness, grace, forgiveness, or patience in those challenging moments. You will be able to access more creativity in problem-solving by being able to think clearly. Perhaps you can recall something you missed in tending to the baby's needs. Perhaps you can come up with a new way to bounce, rock, or stroke the baby. Perhaps you can be present enough to recognize the baby's room is too cold or too hot. Perhaps you remember a lullaby that you want to sing. Perhaps you remember to check on that diaper rash that you forgot about or loosen the diaper or swaddle. There are so many things to think about as a new mother and so much problem-solving to be done. Regulating yourself in the moment helps you feel grounded in your sense as a mother.

Your unique gifts as a mother can meet your child's needs more fully if you can allow them to come through. When I set out to write this book, I read Elizabeth Gilbert's *Big Magic: Creative Living Beyond Fear* no less than 10 times. In the very first chapter, she asks, "Do you have the courage to bring forth the treasures inside you?" Creative living demands the courage. Gilbert's book pertains to various works of art, but it applies to taking care of babies as well. What demands more creativity than the trials and errors of day-to-day living during those first months with a baby? How else do you manage to get everything done while maintaining your sanity? Mothering demands the highest level of creativity, problem-solving, and brain power. Every parent has treasures inside them, their own potential parenting genius ready to be cultivated. I invite you to bring forth your unique treasures.

Model being human. Trust me, my practice is filled with adolescents who aren't allowed to be human and cannot tolerate failures, disappointments, and mistakes. Learn to welcome failure and uncertainty in yourself as a placeholder model for when your babies are old enough to understand. Our children need to allow themselves to be human. Their mothers need to allow themselves to be human too. It is never too early to start this process.

Here are some ways to mother yourself in a moment: Take deep belly breaths. Close your eyes and listen for the most distant sound you can hear. Drink a cup of coffee. Put on an upbeat song and dance or rap to yourself. Take one minute longer to do anything like wash your hands or massage your moisturizer into your face and third eye. Walk more slowly and notice something you like that you see, such as a plant or the shape of a cloud. Call a friend. Take a silly selfie of you flexing your muscles to remind you of your strength (and sense of humor). Eat a piece of chocolate. Drink a warm cup of tea or milk. Eat a pastry. Shave your legs. Buy a lotion or soap with a scent that you like and use it daily. Don't save it for date night or going out. Use it every single day. Paint a picture. Color in a coloring book.

Watch a funny movie. Watch a funny YouTube clip. Write in a journal. Pray. Light a candle. List three things you are grateful for. Go for a bike ride. Go for a walk in the woods. Jump in puddles. Take a deep breath. Walk on the beach. Visualize yourself exercising. Window shop. Take a nap. Allow screentime and take a break. Listen to a motivating book or podcast. Knit something. Take a long shower and lock the door. Cook a delicious meal or snack. Do a yoga pose— child's pose for 30 seconds can restore sleep. Listen to spa music. Stretch. Sing your favorite song at the top of your lungs. Watch a TED Talk. Take up needlepointing. Take your vitamins or medication. Scream into a pillow. Sit outside. Mentally plan a vacation to a destination of your choice, and be specific with the details. Take a break from social media. Unfollow accounts that don't make you feel good. Dry your hair. Make a funny video. Play a board game. Smell your baby's hair. Have a fashion show for yourself. Organize something. Purge your closet. Apply a facial mask. Get a pedicure with an extra five-minute massage. Get some ice cream. Say no to something. Revisit an old hobby. Learn something new. Read a magazine. Take a mental health day. Crochet. Visit the library or bookstore and pick a book. Do a puzzle. Play the *New York Times* Spelling Bee. Listen to an audiobook. Sit in silence. Write a letter to yourself praising something you have done recently. Play. Buy some cozy socks. Have your partner give you a foot massage. Lock yourself in your closet and scroll through funny memes. Set a boundary.

Mothering yourself is not the same thing as treatment, but it can help shift mindset. Mother yourself more.

Matrescence and the Transition to Motherhood

- Focus on your needs first.
- Mothering is regulating your own emotions, and this will help your child regulate their own emotions.
- For example, a counterintuitive, mother-centric approach during a baby's lengthy crying jag would be, "How am I feeling in this moment? Am I feeling powerless, scared, or angry? If so, how can I tend to these emotions first?" By doing this first, you regulate your own emotions, which will allow you to access all the wonderful resources you have (e.g., the abilities to soothe, feed, entertain), then decide what to do in that moment.
- Mothering is making good choices regardless of the outcome.

We must remind ourselves that as mothers, we are caregivers. In psychology, we have made more advances in the field of caregiving research. Motherhood is the ultimate caregiving experience. During my postdoctoral fellowship at the University of Colorado, I focused solely on developing interventions to help caregivers take better care of themselves while taking care of loved ones. The intervention does not involve the dependent patient at all, and caregivers stated that they were grateful to have something only for them.

In caregiver research, biomarkers can indicate the physiological toll caregiving has on the body. For example, telomere length is shortened and is related to more stressful caregiving. Telomeres are casings that simply protect strands of DNA. When cells divide, telomeres are lost. Telomeres are replenished by an enzyme called telomerase. However, chronic stress associated with caregiving can decrease your supply, resulting in cell death or the cell contributing to inflammation. What does this tell us? Many things, but of importance, 1) caregivers must manage their stress to be a better caregiver, and 2) mothers are always caregivers, so the stress of the mother role can be viewed in the same light as that of the caregiver.

It is now known that the better caregivers take care of themselves, the better they can take care of others. Caregivers are also more likely to experience depression, anxiety, and distress. Furthermore, caregivers' mental health can influence patients' mental health. A large body of research promotes this notion that caregivers and the loved ones they care for are interdependent; such that the psychological functioning of the caregiver impacts the patient. For example, caregivers with lower caregiver strain, better mental health status, and greater ability to help patients engage in medical treatment self-care predicted better outcomes for patients, including event-free survival for one year post-treatment in heart failure patients. Psychobiological research is now focusing on how to improve caregivers' quality of life and investigating further the specific patient outcomes that are a result of their caregivers' psychological abilities.

Taking better care of yourself to better care for your baby is counterintuitive. It makes no sense from a biological perspective. Psychologically and in the long term, I argue that the mother's needs are *more* important. We know that a baby's development is most influenced by the mental health of the primary caregiver. This is counterintuitive at birth, as mothers are primed to viscerally respond to a baby's cry, feed them all the time, remove any potential danger—anything that can impact their survival. Mothers are responsible for it all, often not even aware that they are, in fact, neglecting their own needs. Society also places unique stress on mothers. Mothers have never been so isolated yet so observed and judged as they are now. It's challenging for any parent to get their needs fully met during early child-rearing. However, we can do better by working together to listen, respond, and work toward meeting mothers' needs better. Remember, the better you take care of yourself, the better you will be able to take care of your dependents.

In my practice, I see mothers who are depleted. Mothers who are carrying an immense mental load, being pulled in so many directions, and feeling all the postpartum pressures. They are the mothers who seem like everything is fine on the surface as they manage to keep it all together. However, underneath, symptoms of high-functioning depression and anxiety are present. High-functioning anxiety and depression are not recognized as formal diagnoses in our diagnostic manuals. The Harvard School of Public Health calls it "low-grade depression."[25] It is also known as "smiling depression." Carol Landau, professor of psychiatry and medicine at Brown University, states that "it is not a category that appears in the textbooks."[26] Therefore, high-functioning depression and anxiety are often missed by family, friends, and even medical providers. This is another reason why it is imperative to seek consultation from a mental health professional if something feels off.

When assessing high-functioning depression in my patients, I look for loss of motivation, perfectionistic thinking, feeling down at times, feeling irritable, bleak outlooks on the future, and other ways that the patient is suffering but not to the point of interfering with the ability to function in their daily lives. With high-functioning anxiety, I look for busyness, overachievement, perfectionism, rigid and distorted thoughts, difficulty saying no, never feeling good enough, and other clues that indicate things are worse than they seem. Oftentimes, it is those who look like they are calm, cool, and collected who are working the hardest to keep their true feelings hidden. If there is any question, talk to a mental health specialist.

Matrescence and the Transition to Motherhood

- Mothers are the ultimate caregiver. Caregivers are more prone to experience anxiety, stress, and depression.
- You must put on your oxygen mask first before helping others. It is counterintuitive, but in times of stress, anxiety, and depression, dig deeper into treatment and self-care.
- The strongest predictor of childhood well-being is maternal mental health.
- High-functioning depression looks different from clinical depression. Sometimes it is not obvious when a high-functioning mom is suffering. Lying in bed all day is not the way high-functioning depression presents. Look for distorted thinking. Depression is a real medical illness, and you don't need a reason to be depressed.
- High-functioning anxiety looks different from clinical levels of anxiety. Look for perfectionistic thinking, avoidance of failure, irritability, making careless mistakes, or feeling overwhelmed.

5

PREP YOUR MARRIAGE

"People think I'm being catty by saying this—it's like, there were 10 years where I couldn't stand my husband. And guess when it happened? When those kids were little."
—MICHELLE OBAMA

"Dr. Pensak, I can't stand my partner."

This is one of the most common openings in sessions when I work with parents with infants, especially first-time mothers. Nobody is getting their needs met. Everyone is exhausted. Life looks nothing like the way they anticipated it compared to the freedom they had before baby, and it is a huge adjustment. Marital satisfaction plummets post-baby. Read that again. If you are not having the most exciting years of marriage after having a baby, you are having the typical marriage experience in early parenthood. This may come as a shock or disappointment or anywhere in between. One of the most helpful aspects of my job as a clinical psychologist is to inform my patients that their dissatisfaction with their partners, marriage, etc. is, for the most part, within normal limits. I frequently recommend the book *How Not to Hate Your Husband After Kids* by Jancee Dunn because it resonates with many couples' reality of having babies.

Now, of course there are ranges in severity and some couples are suffering more than they should. There are also many ways to improve relationships even within the early parenting phase. Couples therapy can help assess what is typical of this phase and what is not. I am saying this to empower you. Even in this pleasure suck phase of marriage, you can still have a good marriage, arousal, and desire, within reason. Yes, there are practical limits. There is a ceiling as to how good it can get during this early parenthood phase, I assure you.

Regardless of the strain that having a baby can put on a marriage, there are many ways to protect, prevent, and soften the blow. First, it is helpful to have a proactive discussion on the division of labor in the household before the baby comes as well as regular check-ins to discuss how the plan is working, reallocate tasks if necessary, and talk about what is going well. Eve Rodsky, author of *Fair Play*, offers practical examples of how to go through this process. In addition, there is also a Fair Play card deck that includes 100 domestic tasks to discuss and divvy up between partners. It is important to note that when you take responsibility for a card and task, you are taking psychological responsibility for the entirety of the task. This means that the partner responsible has to remember to do the task, execute the task, and be psychologically aware of all components of the task. For example, if a partner agrees to be responsible for emptying the trash, this means that same partner keeps track of the garbage piling up, takes the trash out when it is full, puts another garbage bag in the trash can, and repeats as necessary. It does not count when the other partner prompts the responsible partner to "take out the trash." This defeats the purpose because it places the psychological responsibility of the trash on the partner who does not hold the card, thus adding to the mental load. The goal of the division of tasks is to reduce the mental load. It is important to remember that when you are dividing up the tasks, the division is not about "equal," it is about perceived fairness from both partners. In other words, one partner may hold more cards than the other and still believe it is a fair breakdown of responsibilities.

When I recommend the Fair Play plan to my patients, I specifically tailor my recommendations to each patient because recommending Fair Play without taking into account mental health factors may interfere with successful implementation. When I spoke to Rodsky, she agreed, noting that she is prioritizing training mental health clinicians to disseminate Fair Play. While her program focuses on the task plan, clinicians and individuals need to take the following factors into account when they are considering using Fair Play methods. First, depression and anxiety can distort perception. If one partner is suffering, then everything can feel overwhelming and unfair, thus perpetuating an imbalance of responsibilities. The tasks will not be distributed fairly because nothing will seem fair.

Mom guilt, mom shame, and mom rage, which I will discuss in later chapters, can also interfere with initiating and maintaining Fair Play task division. There are many effective ways to reduce mom guilt. Mothers may feel guilty admitting they need help or they "can't do everything." This is a distorted perception and worth exploring and reducing so that mothers may feel free to delegate tasks. The same is true for mom shame, when mothers can't live up to the "ideal mother" stereotype, which states they should do it all and be self-sacrificing. If they can't meet these standards, they think they are "failing." Mom rage occurs from depletion and being triggered when mothers don't have enough in the tank. It would be a good study to examine if Fair Play has an impact on mom rage. With my patients, I have this discussion often when they report resentment and rage toward their partner. Division of domestic tasks is one of the elements I address when mothers are experiencing mom rage. What mom doesn't feel ragey when the Diaper Genie is full, stinks up the house, and their partner adds another diaper to it without taking it out and replacing the cartridge? In addition, I counsel my patients that when they truly delegate a task, they have to be okay with the dishwasher being loaded backward, or the clothes being folded differently than how you would do it.

Most importantly, and when I think about how Fair Play methods can support the developmental stage of becoming a mother, matrescence, mothers can get lost in the process, often saying "this is not what I expected" due to mental load and household demands. Let's help mothers get back to mothering, which includes the more rewarding and fulfilling parts. This will help mothers reap the benefits of motherhood and nurture the process. Every mother deserves the space to get more pleasure from motherhood. When we reduce the mental load, tedious tasks, monotony, and stress, there is more potential for those moments to occur, enabling mothers to engage in higher-order tasks that challenge and further develop their brains.

Furthermore, because the maternal brain is brilliant, I often think how balancing the division of household labor can nurture maternal brain plasticity in the first two years of motherhood. The early parental brain is primed for new learning, making it an opportune time to learn essential methods for managing a household smoothly. By riding the tidal wave of neuroplasticity, these methods become more integrated in the brain. The maternal brain is responsible for greater problem-solving abilities, mentalizing, creativity, efficiency, and brilliance. When mothers can delegate the more mundane household tasks, this frees up their brain to rise to higher-order tasks. For example, when a mother can tell a family visitor to wash bottles, perhaps she will have more time to take care of herself and further nurture the brilliance emerging by allowing her to have the space for introspection. When you delegate, be very specific in your instructions. For example, say "Go to the grocery store and pick up x, y, and z," or "Take the towels out of the dryer, fold them, and put them away in the linen closet."

Another integral aspect of marriage that changes when you have a baby is intimacy. Unlike the octopus, I am constantly in the process of noticing my own needs. For example, on Mother's Day last year, all I wanted was an hour of alone time, or two or three. Instead, my daughter, as per our usual morning routine, cuddled with me all morning, and even as I took some time to enjoy writing this very passage, she lay next to me with her back leaning against mine. I marveled at the amazing emotional connection we shared and simultaneously craved that space that allowed me to explore my innermost thoughts. My son has been in a "mama" phase lately, so I spent Mother's Day, as I spend most of my extracurricular time, with two need machines *attached to me* until the evening after bedtime. Two dialectical things can be true in mothering: "I love my kids more than anything, and I need time away from them immediately."

My husband, in contrast, always seems to step out of the shower in the evenings, his towel wrapped around his waist, and nuzzles up next to me the second I get a chance to lay my head on the pillow. He is in partner mode while I am still in mother mode. I am impressed by his ability to seamlessly switch from surgeon, to father, to husband, and back 10 times over without skipping a beat. I, on the other hand, want to be suspended in space, no contact with the world around me, my own dark abyss bliss. I need time to reenter my body and feel that I am a woman, a partner, and a sexual being again.

Recently, after a particular touched-out day, I needed to protect some non-touching time for my sanity. I told my husband that after I put the kids to bed, I needed at least 20 minutes during which he does not initiate anything in the form of foreplay. I needed time to transition from the role of need fulfiller to partner to my husband and mother to myself. Sometimes that means my husband and I lie in bed, holding hands while watching nature shows or Bill Maher until we pass out. Sometimes it means more.

Motherhood requires an evolution of how to maintain your relationships, including your marriage. I decided that this is what I needed to be able to meet the needs of our marriage, something that is sacred in my life. When I don't want to be touched or connect with him at the end of a long day, I remind him of the overstimulation and mental load that is likely interfering. I make a direct statement about how much time I may need and that I will consider it again after that time frame. Then I check in with myself to see how I feel after the time has passed. Remember, some days you may need 20 minutes of no touching, some days 20 hours, and some days even five minutes will do.

In general, mystery is one of nature's aphrodisiacs. You know what the opposite of mystery is? Parenthood. This is a good thing for your family but not great for the bedroom. Between those wake and sleep hours, dirty diapers, feeding, laundry, doctor appointments, grocery shopping, drop-offs, pickups, schedule coordination, meal prepping, maybe a shower, work tasks, coffees, and the nonstop day-to-day responsibilities fill your time and are all part of the mental load. After you finally get the baby to sleep and are finished being a feeding, cleaning, nurturing, entertaining machine, you get to retreat to your bed. You turn over and realize there is another need machine next to you, and maybe you both sigh together in exhaustion. Or maybe one of you has less energy and desire because they had to do baby feedings in the middle of the night. Whatever the reason, when your partner gestures to get it on, your mommy brain short-circuits.

A neural pathway that was flooded with parental signals now gets an interrupting signal, expecting a switch to wife brain or sexual partner brain, and cannot comprehend. It is well known that desire and arousal work differently for women compared to men, especially as we age and are in long-term, committed relationships. Men are more likely to get turned on before the act of intimacy and as such are motivated by their arousal to get into the act. Women, on the other hand, need to start the act of intimacy, and then over time and the more they get into it, arousal and desire follow. In other words, many women have to start having sex, settle in to and relax into it, and then desire and arousal will follow. This may, for practical reasons, just take more time than you are used to prior to babies. It may take practice to get into "sexual being" mode more quickly, considering all the baby-related interruptions and psychological preoccupation of tending to a baby's needs.

What this means is that women tend to say yes to intimacy before they feel the arousal. So it is understandable that you say no. Dr. Virginia Sadock, director of the Program in Human Sexuality and Sex Therapy at NYU Medical Center, reported that women are more complicated sexually.[27] In research studies conducted by her lab in which men are hooked up to monitors that measure their arousal, the monitors will show they are aroused when they say they are visually aroused to pornography. However, if you do the same thing with women, even if they say they will be turned on by pornography, some of the monitors will show arousal and some will not. Women also tend to prefer more foreplay in the forms of physical affection, being held, cuddling, and kissing. Men prefer genital stimulation.

It is important to know that your vagina will be dry after you have a baby. When you want to consider sex again, stock up on over-the-counter lubricants. Sex should not be painful. If you are experiencing pain, more than a little discomfort, make an appointment with a perinatal pelvic floor occupational therapist or physical therapist. Make sure they are certified in pelvic floor therapy.

Anxiety, depression, and certain medications like antidepressants and antihistamines can also impact sexual functioning. There are many other barriers to intimacy postpartum, and it's challenging to make intimacy a priority. If you want to say no every time you don't feel like being intimate, that is your decision and I stand by what you decide. I am not saying you always have to say yes when you don't want to. What I am saying is that you may say no because you feel like your desire will show up one day and you'll spontaneously be in the mood next week. What I am educating you on regarding your new mommy brain and arousal system is that arousal typically comes after engaging in intimacy, not before intimacy starts. If you choose to make an effort in this arena, you could start off saying yes as a placeholder for future intimate moments you will enjoy more. Tell your partner you want to start with just holding each other and then go from there.

I just want to emphasize that "next week" you will still be emptying the Diaper Genie, feeling touched out, and cobbling together lunches for daycare at the last minute. You will still get through your day doing all the things. You will likely not feel a yearning for your partner that makes you want to pounce with desire. (If you do experience this, congratulations, you don't need this passage.) It does not mean that the desire won't improve. It will just take effort on your part to go through the motions, allow yourself to settle in to your body, and figure out a way—perhaps by relaxing into your body, cuddling, or sensory massage—to improve intimacy.

There are many cognitive behavioral strategies for improving intimacy that can be applied in the postpartum period when you are ready. You can work with a therapist to help identify your own thoughts and feelings about intimacy after giving birth, as they may have changed. There are also many physical conditions that can influence intimacy. Some common symptoms include pelvic floor dysfunction, vaginismus (involuntary tensing of vagina), and dyspareunia (pain during intercourse). You can engage in pelvic floor rehabilitation, ask your medical provider about creams and lubricants for pain, or use dilators to gradually, comfortably expand the vagina. In addition, some patients feel anxious and depressed related to intimacy, so it is important to talk about your thoughts and feelings with a trained professional. The experience of pain during intimacy can also be influenced by mood. Cognitive behavioral therapy—an evidence-based treatment for sexual dysfunction, pain, depression, and anxiety—can help you shift your thoughts and feelings around intimacy if these conditions are interfering.

You can redefine intimacy for what works in this stage of parenting and every other stage of parenting. In the infancy stage, maybe cuddling is the priority and holding hands while you sleep is the intimacy. Maybe when the baby starts to sleep through the night, you'll have more time and space to consider more physical intimacy. Perhaps on days when you are touched out by your toddler, just lying next to each other while watching a funny movie is enough.

Lower expectations again, and then again. Have conversations about different types of intimacy and each partner's preferences. Create space to connect. Allow the act of intimacy to increase the arousal for intimacy. It is not automatic, so give yourself time. Practice deep breathing. Set different goals. Perhaps the goal of orgasm is too out of reach for the brief window of time before you fall asleep. That's okay. Maybe just feeling your partner lie on top of you or smelling his hair or skin is enough to connect for the time being.

Your pleasure center changes in motherhood. Your arousal and desire change, and that is all to be expected. While there are strategies that can improve intimacy, it is never going to be like the honeymoon phase again. Say goodbye to that phase because it is synonymous with uncertainty. Parenthood and family life require certainty. Mothering requires consistency. Certainty and predictability are NOT aphrodisiacs.

SNAPSHOT

Prep Your Marriage

- Your brain's reward circuit changes when you become a parent. You may not get the same amount of pleasure from the things that used to bring you pleasure. There are incredible highs with parenting and lower lows.
- Certainty is not an aphrodisiac.
- Lower your expectations of what life will be like post-baby.
- Then lower your expectations again.
- Despite these expectations, there are many strategies that can enhance intimacy. Redefine intimacy and what it means to you and your partner (e.g., touching, massage, holding hands, intimate conversation, watching a show, intercourse).
- Revise at any point, as it may change reflective of your little one's developmental stages (e.g., newborn, infancy, toddlerhood).
- To increase arousal and desire in women, women have to spend time in the act and then get aroused. It takes time. Be patient. Feel free to experiment with things that can speed it up (e.g., vibrators or lubricants).
- As mothers, our entire being changes. Our brain, the pathways, the neurotransmitters, our psyches, hormones, relationships, interests, schedules, needs, and pleasures ALL CHANGE.

John Gottman, a renowned couples therapist, describes four major pitfalls in relationships that can lead to demise: criticism, defensiveness, contempt, and stonewalling. Criticism is verbally attacking a partner's character. Defensiveness is claiming to be the victim when faced with confrontation and not taking your partner's perspective into account. Contempt is hateful acts, such as intending to abuse or insult the other person. Finally, stonewalling is pathological avoidance and withdrawal from the relationship. These four concepts are predictors of divorce.

Thankfully, Dr. Gottman provides "antidotes" to each of these notions. For criticism, the antidote is to use "I" statements and acknowledge a positive need. For example, "*I understand you didn't mean to hurt me, but your action made me feel less than. In the future, I would appreciate if you didn't use that language.*" To counter defensiveness, try accepting responsibility. For example, "*That was not my intention, and I see that I hurt you. I apologize. I will correct this tomorrow and make sure it is resolved.*" To rectify contempt, try appreciation. For example, point out your partner's positive qualities and practice gratitude: "*I appreciate you being direct. You are always able to come to me to tell me honestly how you feel. I am so grateful I have a partner that is honest with me.*" Finally, for stonewalling, try taking a break and coming back to discuss the issue with your partner. Try saying, "*I am feeling overwhelmed right now. I want to give this matter the attention it deserves. Would you mind if I go for a walk outside, and when I get back we can sort this out together?*"

Prep Your Marriage

There are four predictors of divorce, according to John Gottman, PhD, renowned couples expert.

- Criticism: Verbally attacking a partner's character.
- Antidote: Use "I" statements and acknowledge a positive need (e.g., "*I understand you didn't mean to hurt me, and your action made me feel less than. In the future, I would appreciate you not using that language.*").
- Defensiveness: Claiming to be the victim when faced with confrontation and not taking partner's perspective into account.
- Antidote: Accept responsibility (e.g., "*That was not my intention, and I see that I hurt you. I apologize.*").
- Contempt: Hateful acts, such as intending to abuse or insult the other person.
- Antidote: Try appreciation and gratitude; be specific (e.g., "*I appreciate you being direct. You are always able to come to me and tell me how you feel. I am so grateful to have a partner that is honest with me.*").
- Stonewalling: Pathological avoidance and withdrawal from the relationship.
- Antidote: Take a break and come back to discuss the issue with your partner (e.g., "*I am feeling overwhelmed right now. I want to give this matter the attention it deserves. I am going to take a break for 30 minutes, and when I come back let's sort this out together.*").

Gottman further suggests a positive-to-negative-experience ratio of approximately five-to-one. In other words, couples should strive for increasing positive experiences in the face of negative experiences, and the goal is around five positive for every one negative. It is not a hard-and-fast rule, but it is based on Gottman's research-driven data. Gottman suggests that this also fills up an emotional bank account. The more positive experiences you have in the bank, the more reserve you have as a couple.

Another way to increase the emotional bank account is by completing "bids." A bid is when your partner turns toward you and bids for your response. Sometimes it is easy to miss bids, but the miss can have a negative impact. So when your partner reaches for your hand, asks how you are doing, or asks you to do something together, say yes more. It's easy to think these small moments don't matter that much when you have all the other things to do. However, in early parenthood, you mostly get small moments. Bread crumbs. Notice, gather, and store them in your cheek because winter *is* coming. It's always just around the corner.

As a reminder, satisfaction decreases dramatically in the first years of parenthood. How can it not? What is there to argue about before babies? Stress feels different after babies are born and there are not enough resources for anyone. Conflict easily occurs. We don't always have to fight, but we do have to find a way to talk about difficult matters. Lack of intimacy, dissatisfaction, disappointments, and challenges are great topics in these early years. Not exactly to resolve, but to hold a space for their importance. Keep talking about the things that are important, and eventually you can figure out how to problem-solve around the issue. Marriage is a series of difficult conversations. If you don't want to have challenging conversations about many of the same important things repeatedly, don't get married.

Prep Your Marriage

- Gottman's five-to-one ratio is good to keep in mind. Try to make five positive experiences for every one negative experience.
- Positive experiences can include anything: watching a funny movie, massaging your partner's feet, holding hands, snuggling, going for a walk together, planning/going on a vacation or date together, trying something new together, playing a game, kissing, being intimate, completing a project together, etc. It doesn't have to be huge to fill the bank.
- Have difficult conversations often.
- Turn toward "bids." Recognize the subtle and overt ways your partner is "turning toward" you and accept bids.
- Say yes more.
- Try small gestures of physical affection.
- Look in your partner's eyes when communicating.
- Try to do small things together.
- Put down the phone and connect.
- In early motherhood, you mostly get small moments. Bread crumbs. Take them, store them, and build up your relationship bank.

PART II

How to Adjust to New Mom Experiences and Emotions

6

BABY BONDING AND THE FIRST LETDOWN

"A mother's heart breaks a million ways in her lifetime."
—ASHLEY AUDRAIN, *THE PUSH*

With my first baby, I remember thinking, "I know I love her more than anything, but do I *feel* I love her? How will I know? What is this supposed to feel like?" It is certainly depicted in the movies that a mother just coos over her baby and falls in love immediately. In those early months, I wasn't gaga over my baby or gaga over the process. I felt shame and fear that something was wrong with me. I knew I wanted to take care of Jordan and I knew more than anything that I wanted to be a mother and her mother. I just didn't *feel* it.

A leading maternal researcher, Pilyoung Kim, PhD, has been studying fMRI scans of mothers to better understand maternal brain development. She posits that in the first several months postpartum, there is a wealth of new learning, from changing diapers, to breastfeeding, to learning sensitive ways to respond to the baby. Biology helps us become attracted to our baby and feel an immense sense of importance related to taking care of the baby. But it is very important to recognize that this does not mean that you feel bonded to your baby immediately. Bonding is a process that takes place over time. I ask my patients if they have ever found it easy or immediate to feel emotionally bonded to something that just sleeps, poops, and cries in the early months. Their likely answer is no. Kim further explains that it's not so much the bond as it is the realization of the responsibility and profound significance of taking care of your baby that occurs in a very core, foundational way. I reflected and thought, *Isn't this how most great relationships start? Set to simmer and let it develop over time. Besides, the beginning of a new relationship is all projection anyway.*

Society's unrealistic expectations imply that mothers need to know how to do everything for the baby immediately. That they need to love and feel bonded to their baby on day one. We agree that it would help mothers if society lowered their expectations. Modern-day mothers have more access to filtered images and content that hide the realities of motherhood. The images of a baby dressed in couture and captions that follow—"I am so in love, she's perfect"—are just snapshots of a blip in time followed by consecutive moments of dirty diapers, fussing, and exhausted parents. Nobody wants to share those images though.

Kim explains, "When a baby is born, a mother develops. Mothers are constantly making adjustments depending on the personality of the baby and their experiences with their baby. It's bidirectional. There is strong evidence that the emotional bond between mother and baby is gradual and adapts and changes over time. Be patient and trust that you will get there and develop a strong emotional attachment."

A thought experiment I like to try with mothers who worry about baby bonding is to ask them, "Have you ever felt particularly bonded to a *blueberry* (insert fruit/vegetable/inanimate object here)?" Typically, their response is no. Yet, here we are as mothers, downloading those mobile apps that tell us what size our baby is week to week and compare its size to a piece of granola or a tampon or something ridiculous. It helps if you put the worries about baby bonding into perspective and remind yourself, with a little humor, that bonding takes place over time.

Baby Bonding and the First Letdown

- Baby bonding takes place over time; it is not immediate. There is strong evidence that the emotional bond between mother and baby is gradual and adapts and changes over time.
- Don't try to change your feelings. Accept that you may not feel bonded to your baby. Be patient and kind to yourself. This causes a feeling on top of a feeling, which can further complicate things and contribute to feelings of depression and anxiety.
- There are many things we cannot control in early parenthood. Worrying about things that are out of your control is called unproductive worry.
- It is your job to protect your brain.

In early motherhood, there is always something ready to teach us more about what we cannot control. As early mothers and parents, our main responsibility is protecting our babies and preventing them from getting hurt. We are primarily responsible for their safety. Even with the best intentions and tightly controlled environments, we must accept the reality that there are still things we cannot control. The first letdown is the realization that we cannot control our bonding feelings toward our baby. We must trust that they will develop over time. This letdown is followed by copious daily reminders of other things we cannot control in motherhood, like when our baby doesn't latch, or is allergic to cow's milk, or has a tongue-tie, or if the baby is breech and you need an emergency C-section when you wanted to deliver vaginally, or when your baby spikes a fever on the same day you have that meeting with a new client, or you have to cancel plans with your best friend for the fifth time because of the daily rotating virus, teething pain, sleep regression, or weird rash thing you need to tend to immediately.

When I meet with my patients who speak about their disappointments regarding baby bonding, I remind them of the emotion-focused strategies to help them cope. First, I remind them to fake it until they make it. The baby can't tell if you are faking a smile, or a coo, or a hug, or affection—you might have to fake it at first until the real feelings come through. Not falling in love with your baby immediately falls in the category of a shadowloss. A shadowloss is a loss that occurs in life but not of life. For example, you may feel a shadowloss when you are disappointed in the sex of your baby, in your baby's temperament, in a birth complication, or family members not being as helpful as you had hoped. There are many other types of shadowlosses. It is important to grieve those losses. Grieving time, which is similar to worry time, can help. Set a timer for 10 minutes per day and allow yourself to process that loss within those boundaries. Follow up the grieving time with a pleasant activity. Repeat once per day as needed.

Another emotion-focused coping strategy for when new mothers feel anxious, panicked, and pressured about not bonding is repeating a mommy mantra in their head. Some mantras that I have not mentioned yet include "This is not an emergency even though it feels like one," or "I am enough," or "I am safe, my baby is safe." You can come up with your own and repeat it in your head to slow things down when you feel overwhelmed. If you cannot come up with a mommy mantra of your own, consider repeating the number one in your head. Your mind will want to wander, which is common. Just notice your thoughts and bring it right back to the mantra.

In early motherhood, it often feels like things move so fast. I found this especially to be the case with having a baby and a toddler. When I become overwhelmed with all the things that need to get done, I slow down. It's another one of those counterintuitive strategies. You're probably wondering why I would slow down when I need to speed up to get everything completed. Trust me, it is helpful to slow things down, to slow yourself down. The problem isn't all the things (although maybe sometimes it is), the problem is your body's response to all the things. When you slow your body's response, all the things will feel more manageable, you will be able to think more clearly and efficiently, and all the things will actually be more manageable. When my mind is racing, I physically move my body in slow motion, one step at a time, and focus on my breath.

It should be noted that there is not a one-size-fits-all approach to coping. Plus, a strategy that works for you in one moment might not work in the next. Remember to create a coping card, which lists the strategies that typically work for you. Take a picture of the card and keep it on your phone. That way it's with you at all times. Keep a copy on your nightstand and any other convenient area. This way, if you are feeling overwhelmed, you don't have to think about coming up with the strategies. You can just run down the list.

I advise my patients to match the level of anxiety they are feeling to the strength of the coping strategy. If a patient is starting to feel a little bit anxious, I instruct her to start with deep breathing. If, however, a patient is midspiral, obsessing and ruminating about something very fearful, I advise her to take a book, move line by line, and circle every other a on the page. Or to dunk her head in ice water, then repeat.

Besides the broad emotion-focused and problem-solving coping strategies, I also need to speak about the mom-specific coping strategies that I teach my patients. The first mom-specific category is overstimulation. With the hands-on phase of early parenthood, moms often feel touched out and overstimulated. After a long evening of bath time, playtime, cuddling, and bedtime routines, I regularly tell my husband I need some alone time after I get into bed. This time helps me reenter my body and protect myself from having to be touched yet again. With a baby, it's hard to get that physical space. But with your partner, you can assert yourself.

Overstimulation is a common problem for mothers. I advise mothers to look for ways to reduce stimulation when necessary. Some common strategies are to turn off any television, music, and background noise. Disconnect from your phone. Sometimes this means putting your phone in another room. Sometimes it means deleting applications from your phone entirely and taking a break.

Try experimenting with soothing sounds—nature, white noise, or soft music. Noise-canceling headphones can be used as well. Make a cozy, quiet space in your home. Communicate with your partner and family, and set boundaries so that you can use this space when you need to. Do mindfulness and breathing exercises.

Here, I would like to leave you with three overstimulation strategies that I came up with during the pandemic, when I was not able to leave my house. These strategies still serve me well when I am home with my little ones and need to reduce stimulation. When I am feeling particularly touched out, I get in bed and put the pillows around me to create a cocoon of softness. I then lower my head down on my pillow and pull the covers up so that I am nestled comfortably. I tell my husband not to ask me any questions and pretend I am not here. In this space, I then read something nonactivating to myself. Bonus points if you add noise-canceling headphones in the mix—they are a game changer and pure bliss.

Try taking an escapist shower or a bath. In the shower, stand under the stream of water. Submerge yourself so that just your nose is peeking out to breathe. The water then surrounds your head and ears, blocking out any extraneous noise. Focus on the sounds of the water. Take deep, restorative breaths. Let yourself stay there and imagine you are standing under a waterfall in a tropical place. Repeat. Water is healing. Marine biologist and author Wallace J. Nichols wrote a book, *Blue*

Mind: The Surprising Science That Shows How Being Near, In, On, or Under Water Can Make You Happier, Healthier, More Connected, and Better at What You Do. I support the meditative and healing properties of water.

You've heard the common advice "just add water" referring to a way to shift the energy with little ones. This works for adults too. When I am finished bathing my littles, I have my husband take them out and tell him to close and lock the door. I turn the lights out, except for a dim bath light. Then I turn the bath faucet on and submerge myself on my back under water except for my face. The faucet of water creates enough noise to block out any phantom baby cries and, like the shower, creates a nice, soothing pocket of space in which to lie and breathe. The water obscures the background noise, which allows you to get sensory space. Repeat.

As I mentioned before, in every situation there are things in your control and out of your control. It's up to you to tease apart what is actually out of your control and match it with a proper emotion-focused technique. For the aspects that are truly in your control, there is problem-solving coping. Problem-solving coping simply means finding a solution for the situation that is in your control. An example of something that is in your control includes seeking professional help and treatment.

For me, when I am overstimulated, I rely on emotion-focused coping strategies. I paint. I play. I do crafts and read books. I simplify my life. I focus on the present. There is no better tool to bring you into the present than a baby cooing at you and a three-year-old toddler vying for your attention. I smelled my baby's hair. I walked outside, noticing any aspect of nature, like the shapes of the leaves on the trees or the new wildflowers in a neighbor's garden. I planted a garden of tomatoes, cucumbers, peppers, zucchini, strawberries, three types of basil, mint, parsley, and cilantro, and I create meals out of what crops up. These are ways that I protect my brain.

I also protect my brain by managing my mental health, which, for me, has included taking prescription medication. Every morning, I dance to my bathroom counter and excitedly open my prescription of 10mg fluoxetine (i.e., generic Prozac). I hold the bottle up in the mirror as the character Karen from the sitcom *Will and Grace* would hold her dirty martini up and proclaim, "Thank you for coming." Prescribing medication is out of the scope of my practice, but if you really are having trouble coping and nothing seems to help, consider consulting a healthcare professional who is a licensed prescriber who can evaluate your condition and determine whether prescription medication is appropriate for you.

I am especially grateful for my prescription when I am reminded of the challenges of baby bonding; a new COVID variant surge; a humanitarian crisis, such as Russia invading Ukraine; a headline stating, "World's scientists say disastrous climate change is here"; women's rights being taken away; another school shooting; or my toddler suffering from transient synovitis, a benign but scary symptom of viral infection where your little one's legs become immobilized and he screams in pain from no apparent cause. I remind myself what is in my control, what isn't, and lean in to my strategies for coping with uncertainty and problem-solving effectively to steady my pace while feeling rattled in early motherhood.

For Every New Motherhood Challenge

Ask yourself:

Is this in my control?

If YES:
Problem-Solving Coping

If NO:
Emotion-Focused Coping

Problem-Solving Coping Strategies

- Find a practical solution
- Actively solve the problem, if it can be solved

Emotion-Focused Coping Strategies

- 5, 4, 3, 2, 1 Mindfulness
- Deep breathing relaxation exercises
- Distraction (call a friend, watch a funny show, read, listen to music, Go line by line and circle every other "a" on a newspaper, magazine, or book page)
- Dunk your head in a bowl of ice water
- Exercise
- Crafts
- Repeat a mantra

  - "It doesn't have to be perfect to be okay."
  - "This is not an emergency, even though it feels like one."
  - "I am safe, my baby is safe."

Tools to Overcome Overstimulation for Emotion-Focused Coping

- Remove stimuli from environment
- Turn off television, lights, phone, background noise
- Try creating a cocoon of softness in your bed
- Use noise-canceling headphones
- Just add water, escapist shower or bath

7

THE DOUBLE-DOWN METHOD TO MANAGE MOM GUILT

"Between stimulus and response there is a space. In that space is our power to choose our response. In our response lies our growth and our freedom." —VIKTOR FRANKL

It was 3 AM when Max's cry startled me awake, reminding me that, as a mom, there is no need for an alarm clock. I headed down the hallway to Max's room, ready to rock him back to sleep. But my open arms and gentle "Maxi" voice was met with more intense cries of protest. I picked him up and tried to soothe him to no avail. I felt his head, no temperature. I smelled his diaper, no poop. My husband came in the room and said, "I'll take him" as he gestured for me to get some sleep. No doubt, he was just trying to be helpful. Almost immediately after my husband held him, Max's cry quieted and he rested his head on his shoulder.

I wanted to disappear.

I walked back to our room, crawled under the covers, and pulled them over my head.

At the time, I was beginning to think about sending Max to daycare so I could spend more time working instead of just stealing time when Mike could watch him and during Max's regular nap schedule.

Strike that. I lied. I had already made the decision to send Max to daycare and give up the special "Max and Mommy" weekdays we'd had for the past six months.

I lay awake in bed feeling terribly guilty. Had I made a mistake? He didn't even want me to comfort him. Surely I had failed as a mother. My instinctive mom guilt reaction made me try to think of a solution. I know, I'll just put off daycare and keep him home longer. *This will give me time to win him back.* If I was honest with myself though, I had already thought this decision through.

I purposefully chose to send him to daycare because I needed more time for me. My practice was thriving, but I was squeezing too many patients into too few hours. I wanted more time to write and exercise and paint and breathe, alone, in my house, with no background baby noises as a constant soundtrack. But my mom guilt reeled.

Mom guilt is distorted and has no productive function. I take a counterintuitive response to mom guilt with my patients and also try to do this for myself. Instead of listening to my mom guilt and giving in, I root down further. This is because when we are feeling worse moodwise we tend to have more frequent experiences of mom guilt. Also, if we listen to mom guilt and obey what it commands us to do, we are likely sacrificing our own needs. Then we'll feel even worse, thus increasing the likelihood of more mom guilt. My antidote to mom guilt is to double down and lean in.

To double down on mom guilt is to do the thing that is making you feel guilty—to go to work, to that exercise class, to that meeting, to that social engagement, and then to even add more, such as adding on a scenic drive to the engagement, or a new outfit that makes you feel better in your body, or a coffee to perk up, or extra stretching and time to decompress after a workout. Ask yourself how you can make this more enjoyable, pleasurable, or meaningful.

Another example to illustrate the double-down method is a common experience in early motherhood. Many moms feel guilty going back to work. I say, go back to work and immerse yourself in a new project. Sometimes when we go back to work, we are physically there but mentally still home with our baby. Guilt is one of the ways we are still home with our babies, and this impedes our ability to get the benefits of the activity we are engaged in. Work then becomes solely a drain on our resources instead of helping us refill our cup. Taking on a new, creative, fulfilling, and productive project can help us feel better moodwise, give us more confidence, and renew something that has been on the back burner for months or years. Often the thing that is bringing you the mom guilt is the thing that you need to be doing. This is not to say you have to double down every time you feel a twinge of mom guilt, and it is also permission to double down more often. To double down means to strengthen your commitment to that action. That's right, repeat after me: I will double down on mom guilt. In regard to my mom guilt related to daycare, I followed through with my decision.

To explain the double-down method another way, in blackjack, a double down means you double your bet in the middle of a hand in return for only one extra card. It's a way to increase your payout (your reward). At the blackjack table, you indicate that you want to double down by taking your pointer finger and tapping it down on the table. To emphasize that you are doubling down on mom guilt in the moment, you can make a gesture with your pointer finger and tap a surface in front of you twice. If needed, tap harder to disrupt the pull of mom guilt thoughts. This gesture is meant to snap you out of your mom guilt thoughts. With perseverative thoughts, another tactic is to snap a hair elastic on your wrist to jolt you out of your thoughts. This gesture communicates with your brain by jolting your intention elsewhere and changing the channel of mom guilt in your brain.

When I work with my patients with mom guilt, I look at frequency, severity, and duration. How often are you having mom guilt? How long does the mom guilt last? Are they fleeting thoughts or incessant ruminations that lead to tears and behavior changes? Does mom guilt drive decision-making with your baby? Do you feel guilty as you head out with your girlfriends, then quickly adjust and enjoy a night out? Or are you constantly checking your phone to see if your partner texted about the baby or to watch the Nest camera?

A thought-provoking study by Georgia Constantinou and colleagues examined mom guilt. The results indicated that the most common reported themes of mom guilt—"breastfeeding difficulties, essentialism/responsibility, division/depletion, and connection"[28]— pertained to the "motherhood myth." This is the notion that a mother should be the one primarily responsible for the health and well-being of the baby. These unreasonable expectations have been pervasive in the media and in mommy culture for decades. Ultimately, the motherhood myth contributes to resentment, anger, anxiety, stress, and feeling unsuccessful as a mother when reality does not live up to the idyllic representation.

The authors of the Constantinou review describe that mothers respond to the ideal by engaging in what is called "intensive mothering" to try to adhere to the mothering standards put forth by society. The ideal is perfection, which sets unreasonably high expectations and leads mothers to feel ashamed and guilty when they fall short.

Within the concept of intensive mothering, the motherhood myth and idealized mothering messaging assume the mother alone is responsible for the baby's overall well-being, safety, and development. The article goes on to summarize the main parenting concepts that fall under the umbrella of intensive parenting: essentialism, fulfillment, stimulation, child-centered, and challenging. Essentialism refers to the mother being the vital caregiver. Fulfillment is defined as caregivers being fulfilled only by that role and discounts any negative feelings or experiences in parenthood. Stimulation stipulates that the parents primarily engage with young ones, with the dominant goal of cognitive and intellectual stimulation. Child-centered refers to the baby being the center of their parents' universe and the point around which their lives orbit. Challenging is described as the notion that taking care of a baby is rigorous and exhausting.

What was most revealing in the thematic analyses were the actual statements reported throughout the articles that they systematically reviewed. The quotes by mothers demonstrate the themes mentioned previously. Some of the most commanding statements included: "I feel responsible for every cell of his little body" (essentialism/responsibility). Another: "Well, I just had no idea how painful it is in the first two weeks and how difficult it is. Nobody tells you! . . . I mean I read books and books about pregnancy and labor. . . . [P]eople talk about latch and people talk about soreness, but that's about it. I mean, it's painful! Breastfeeding is very hard. It's not the most natural thing in the world. I mean it is natural, but it doesn't just easily happen. We have to work at it" (breastfeeding difficulties). Also: "When he was nursing, right after this, right after when I finally gave in, and he was sobbing and nursing at the same time because he was just so upset. And, I don't remember, I think I almost cried. And I felt it in my heart" (connection). Another telling statement was: "I felt guilty for wanting to do other things than take care of my baby because she needs me so much. How selfish of me to want to be productive instead of take care of this helpless child" (division/depletion).

All these statements represent internal guilt feelings when the experience of motherhood is in disagreement with the idealized version of motherhood dictated by "cultural laws" (i.e., the motherhood myth). It is integral to help mothers free themselves of comparing themselves to an ideal that does not actually exist. The authors highlight the importance of validating mothers' authentic experiences in this transition.

The Double-Down Method to Manage Mom Guilt

- Mom guilt is distorted and has no productive function.
- Root down further and double down on mom guilt.
- The main contributors of mom guilt most commonly experienced pertain to the "motherhood myth": breastfeeding difficulties, essentialism/responsibility, division/depletion, and connection.
- **The motherhood myth** establishes an unrealistic ideal and prompts moms to engage in "intensive mothering," trying to adhere to standards put forth by society, culture, and media. It assumes the mother alone is primarily responsible for a baby's overall well-being and safety.
- **Breastfeeding difficulties** are common. Fed is best. Try to be kind to yourself and remain flexible.
- **Essentialism/responsibility** refers to the faulty notion that the mother is the only vital caregiver. However, the biological mother is not the only person who can fulfill this role.
- **Division/depletion** refers to fulfillment as the false narrative that the primary caregiver is fulfilled solely by their caregiving role. Mothers who are fulfilled in general and by various roles and responsibilities are better able to serve others and take care of others' needs.
- **Connection** is the desire to be bonded to your baby. Bonding takes place over time. Be patient and kind to yourself.

It is imperative to reduce maternal guilt. Indeed, research indicates maternal guilt is associated with anxiety and depression. In another study, the greater symptom frequency and severity of mom guilt is associated with more negative language and more self-associated responsibility for children's challenging emotions. In other words, moms who took responsibility and blamed themselves for their developing little one's challenging emotions experienced increased depressive symptoms. It is unclear which comes first, the chicken or the egg. Fixating on mom guilt can make you feel more depressed. Depression can also make you focus more on thoughts and feelings associated with self-blame and mom guilt. That is why, conceptually, it makes sense to assess mom guilt as a symptom presentation of what may be going on underneath and not necessarily what the mom guilt is telling you in your mind.

We cannot cure mom guilt. The push-pull of motherhood is real. Often we cannot solve the mom guilt dilemma. It's difficult to win, knowing that we have competing demands. However, the goal is not to win, per se. Instead, we can turn down the volume of punishing thoughts and self-torture. You are allowed to focus on yourself. You are a permanent caregiver. You need breaks, outlets, and psychological freedom. And your dependents will be better off the better you take care of yourself in healthy ways. The more you double down on mom guilt, the more you will reap the benefits of the activities you enjoy and improve mood, in turn reducing the "symptom" of mom guilt.

Brené Brown, PhD, an internationally recognized researcher and author on themes of guilt and shame, has published widely on the topic. She discusses the difference between guilt and shame, explaining that guilt is thinking we did something bad, while shame is thinking we are bad. I'll dig deeper into mom shame in the next chapter. In terms of mom guilt, there's no shortage of reasons to feel guilty about something we potentially did that was "bad"—not breastfeeding, getting help with the baby, allowing screen time, packaged purées, plastic toys, formula feeding, leaving on that work trip, forgetting a doctor appointment, and deciding not to do that fourth mommy-and-me class.

Here's some good news to cope with the common experience of mom guilt. Guilt happens when we regret something we did or did not do. It's also an opportunity for repair, which is essential for developing relationships, which is what you're doing with your baby. Ask yourself, if you didn't feel guilt, would you feel motivated to repair? Look at it as an opportunity to learn and model how to reconnect. These are essential life and relationship skills.

My patient, Janelle, frequently talks about her fractured relationship with her mother. Her mother never admitted she did anything wrong, never apologized. Never took the time to reconnect. Janelle was left with conflicting feelings about her own mothering, not knowing when or how to repair. While it was clear from my patient's description that her mother was not psychologically equipped for insight or introspection, I informed Janelle, that she, as a mother, is very capable of repair and thus able to break the cycle. She has the power to take her own guilt and make use of it.

Becoming a mother not only allows you to determine how you want to mother, but it also may bring up complicated feelings about how you were mothered. I often hear from my patients that they grapple with their own childhood experiences and relationships with their mothers more since becoming mothers themselves. Integral to the transition to becoming a mother is to heal your pain about your experience with your own mother. If you lost your mother; if your mother did not meet your needs; if your mother is physically there but not emotionally available to you; if there are mental health, substance abuse, or other circumstances that prevented your mother from nurturing you, you may have a mother wound. It is important to grieve the mother you never had, the mother you wanted, and the loss that you have incurred. In addition, you can use grieving time for any loss or experience you missed out on in pregnancy and postpartum. For example, if you had a birth plan and the delivery experience did not go as planned (as it often does not), grieve the loss of that ideal.

As a psychologist, it has become much more evident to me that every patient is talking about their "mother" or lack thereof during session. I frequently reflect, what is this patient asking for or not asking for in this session? What needs to be mothered? Many of us do not get the mothering we deserve. No matter what, every mother is imperfect and will not be able to provide everything. No one person can do everything. Even when you get solid mothering, becoming a mother yourself will illuminate ways in which different types of mothering impact development—yours and theirs.

Part of becoming a mother involves making peace with how you were or were not mothered. It is no longer helpful to focus energy on trying to mend, fix, repair, or restore any lack of mothering with the past. Instead, it is much more useful, productive, and rewarding to focus that energy on mothering in the present: mothering yourself in a way in which you may have missed and mothering your baby. To heal the mother wound and break the cycle, don't try to fix the past. It's focusing forward. It's giving what you have not been given. In the words of Michelle Obama, when they go low, you find the strength within and you go high. This is the work.

The Double-Down Method to Manage Mom Guilt

- After becoming a mother, you have a much more nuanced understanding of how mothering implicitly impacts you.
- Many of us do not get the mothering we deserve. Ask yourself what needs to be mothered in you.
- When you become a mother (or before), try to make peace with how you were and were not mothered. Channel that energy into taking care of your baby.
- Healing the mother wound is focusing forward, not trying to fix the past.
- **Practice acts of self-love.** Try therapy, compensatory strategies, seeking surrogates, managing your mental health, and self-care. These are skills to mother yourself in ways you may have not been mothered. Loving yourself more enables you to give more to your children.
- **Do something "a little different."** Do something different from what your parents would have done to you in a similar situation, and do something different from what you feel like doing (e.g., if you feel anger and then want to yell, take a beat and try whispering). Over time, these smaller, more manageable steps will build and lead to more resiliency.
- **Make time for mother wound grieving.** For any loss of a mother or mothering, set a timer for 10 minutes no more than once daily to grieve and mourn that loss. Cry, mourn, get angry, write a letter for yourself, and express how you feel. When the timer is up, go do something else. If a wound reminder pops up during the day outside that grieving time window, make a note of it and tell yourself, "I am not going to think about this now. I will think about it during my mother wound grieving time."

In regard to my own mom guilt, I doubled down. The problem was not that Max did not want me to soothe him and preferred my husband. The problem was my mom guilt response. Mom guilt can also be a symptom of not having enough of your needs met. The very appearance of my mom guilt meant that I needed to fill my cup more. I needed to nurture myself and, if I did, if I were working with a full cup, I would be able to brush off that late-night scenario with Max as the nonexistent problem that it was. The very fact that I went to my dark place was a sign that I needed to take care of myself more, and this had nothing to do with Max.

I sat with my mom guilt and made the decision to honor myself. I did not get rid of the mom guilt. In fact, when I dropped Max off at daycare, he clung to me and begged not to go in. I bawled in the car in the parking lot. The point is, I did not try to relieve my mom guilt *before* deciding to go through with my decision. If I waited until my mom guilt was relieved, I would still be spending my days with him until he left for college, planning "Max and Mommy special days."

With time, I was able to tend to my needs more while meeting the demands of my professional work. The mom guilt lessened. It wasn't that Max ended up adjusting to daycare or that he never demonstrated preference for his father again because he does still prefer his father at times and he did in fact adjust quickly to daycare. Now, because I am less stressed and more fulfilled in my work and creative outlets, I can be a better mother to him. I can appreciate my husband's bond with Max and recognize it for the asset that it is. This is counterintuitive. This is the double-down approach to maternal guilt. Dig your heels in and take care of your own needs first. This is the best for you, your family, and your baby.

Another antidote to mom guilt is to keep in mind that, as mothers and parents, we are playing the long game. We will be parents for a very long time. There are abundant opportunities to tend to our dependents' needs in our lifetimes, and not just during the baby stage.

If we come from a place of psychological abundance versus scarcity, we can trust that there will be plenty of opportunities to take care of them and we don't have to cling so hard to "perfection" in the one that is present today.

Not long after daycare started, Max entered a "mommy phase." I can now proudly say I am currently *both* of my children's preferred caregiver, and I am exhausted. I am constantly required to masterfully meet both of my little ones' needs simultaneously, which is impossible and not without some amateur wrestling moves and magician-like distraction. The mommy hands are quicker than the baby and toddler eyes. If I would have continued to sacrifice my needs, Max may still have gotten to the mommy phase, and I may have interpreted that as a result of me spending more time with him when, in fact, the opposite was true. Perhaps by fulfilling my own needs first, I was able to be more present in the more limited time we had together. Or maybe it was just that developing littles go through phases of preferences, and it's nothing to take too personally. Regardless, it took every bone in my body to root down and declare that I was putting mommy first. As a result, I feel much more fulfilled and inspired, which benefits my own psyche, regardless of whom Max may prefer.

Here are some examples of common maternal guilt phrases and how to reframe them with more adaptive thoughts. When you are having mom guilt, feel free to use these as a guide to reframe your own distorted thoughts.

Mom Guilt Says: I feel guilty leaving my baby while I go out.
Healthy Reframe: *It is important for my baby to learn that I will leave and always come back.*

Mom Guilt Says: I do not like the way my babysitter/relative/spouse/ does things with my baby, so I should just do it.
Healthy Reframe: *It is important for my baby to learn and adapt to*

how other people do things because not everyone in the world will do things like mommy.

Mom Guilt Says: The caregiver is not paying enough attention to my baby, and I feel guilty making my baby attend childcare.
Healthy Reframe: *It is important for my baby to be exposed to and inter-act with different types of people. This is one of those opportunities.*

Mom Guilt Says: I feel guilty spending time at work/with friends/doing a hobby, etc.
Healthy Reframe: *It is important that my baby grow up with a mommy who has a big life and life outside them. This way my baby can learn that, when they grow up, it is okay for them to have a life outside mommy.*

Mom Guilt Says: I feel guilty that I expressed anger toward my baby or with my partner/family member/other child.
Healthy Reframe: *It does not have to be perfect to be okay. I can find an opportunity to repair and reconnect by holding, soothing, feeding, reading to, or singing to my baby. I can figure out other ways to reconnect with the other person as well.*

Mom Guilt Says: I feel guilty that I forgot to pack my baby's pacifier, blanky, bottle, extra clothes, or favorite stuffed animal.
Healthy Reframe: *My baby will not die from discomfort.*

Mom Guilt Says: I feel guilty that I do not spend as much time with my second baby as I did when I had my first baby. The older sibling got so much more of my undivided attention.
Healthy Reframe: *This is why birth order matters. It is not a bad thing, and it is a thing. I am not an endless resource. I have limits. Eventually my baby will grow into a child who will learn about limits.*

Mom Guilt Says: I feel guilty for having negative feelings toward my baby.

Healthy Reframe: *I am human and have human feelings. I am a model for my baby to allow the full breadth of my experience as a human and will demonstrate compassion and acceptance toward myself.*

Mom Guilt Says: I feel guilty for not liking/not being able/not wanting to breastfeed.

Healthy Reframe: *There is not a one-size-fits-all approach to taking care of babies. I have preferences, my baby will have preferences, and that is okay.*

Mom Guilt Says: I feel guilty that I feel ambivalent about motherhood.

Healthy Reframe: *Ambivalence is the hallmark experience of motherhood.*

Mom Guilt Says: I feel guilty that I don't like the infant stage.

Healthy Reframe: *The infancy stage is incredibly demanding. Lots of mothers have different preferences for different stages of development. There is no right or wrong. You may like the next stage or later stages more.*

The Double-Down Method to Manage Mom Guilt

- When mothers do not feel validated in their authentic experiences of motherhood, guilt and shame can result.
- Guilt is thinking *you did something bad.*
- Shame is thinking *you are bad.*
- Guilt can be an opportunity to reconnect, which is an essential relationship skill.
- Lean in to and double down on mom guilt, which can be a symptom of not having enough of your needs met. It will pass over time.
- Also, if you are depressed or anxious, you may be more likely to fixate on mom guilt thoughts.
- As you feel better, you will be better able to let go of mom guilt thoughts.
- Remember, you are playing the long game with your baby. View opportunities through a lens of psychological abundance versus scarcity. There will be abundant opportunities to tend to their needs throughout their lifetime.

8

SOFTEN ON MOM SHAME

> "If you put shame in a petri dish, it needs three ingredients to grow exponentially: secrecy, silence, and judgment. If you put the same amount of shame in the petri dish and douse it with empathy, it can't survive."
>
> —BRENÉ BROWN, PHD

I believe all mothers have the power to cultivate the mother they want to be. Mothers can figure anything out if they can understand how to get out of their own way. Shame is a barrier that gets in the way. The problem is, mothers are getting super frustrated and asking for practical advice, what to say, what to do, the perfect schedule, the perfect strategy. Those can all help, but we neglect to remind them to work on themselves in that moment so they can build resiliency and work on cultivating their own solutions or just tolerating the disappointment, the frustration, the imperfect mother-baby moment. If we neglect to teach mothers this skill, they can start a vicious cycle of always looking outward for solutions when, really, their superpowers are underneath, I am sure of it. We need to help them access them.

Jordan was born premature and I battled to breastfeed her. It's the messaging that was passed down, that "babies will eat when they're hungry," with the critical "you're making this too hard on yourself, it's a natural process," juxtaposed with the pediatrician firmly instructing me that she needs to eat every three hours, around the clock, with no margin for error. The battles with nipple guards, the football versus cradle holds, the stroking of her cheek to keep her awake through her premature and jaundice-caused lethargy, and the tears of worry when she skipped a middle-of-the-night feeding after my efforts proved futile. If you spend two hours on one feeding, that leaves one hour until the next feeding. As a first-time mother, the most important thing in the early months was to keep my baby alive, and I understood that to be achieved primarily by breastfeeding. All of this, coupled with new mom anxiety, was a lot to manage.

In those wee hours, blurry eyed and blurry brained from lack of sleep, there seemed to be no more time to problem-solve, to be flexible, to let it play out and wait for my baby to eat when she *feels* hungry as I had been instructed by the mothers before me. I took matters into my own hands and pumped to resolve uncertainty, to help me get more sleep, and to nurture my mental health. That seemed like a win even when, in fact, I felt like I had lost the battle with being able to naturally breastfeed. I tried to focus on the satisfaction of seeing Jordan drink an entire bottle and felt like I was ultimately winning the war.

The "natural processes in motherhood" are actually not natural at all. Maternal instinct is a myth. Breastfeeding often comes with challenges. Motherhood is more about trial and error than anything else. It is on-the-job learning—learning your baby, learning yourself, and learning a million new things you've never had to do before. The myth of "instinct" is really tuning in to your baby's needs based on the amount of time you spend interacting, caring for, and getting to know them. This happens over time and continues throughout their lifetime. It does not magically appear on day one.

When we feel like we are lacking in something maternal, such as the faulty notion of "instinct," shame can ensue. Shame can be a side-eyed glance from another mom on the playground pulling out a nonplastic container of homemade, hidden-vegetable, organic muffins as you scrounge the bottom of your purse for an old pack of goldfish for a snack. It's the baby who doesn't sleep through the night, or doesn't latch immediately, or is colicky, and you think it's all your fault. It's in the nonorganic formula, or a forgotten tummy time session, or a day when you couldn't even shower, or a messy house, or a developmental delay. It's in the late pickup, the raised voice, the missed opportunity to play classical music to your baby in the womb, the C-section, the epidural, the choice to wean from breastfeeding, or the baby weight. It's the "I don't feel bonded to my baby, what's wrong with me?" Or feeling incredibly proud that you got your baby and toddler out the door at the same time—only to focus on the forgotten diaper bag.

Shame is taking those sounds and making them signals when in fact they are just noise. It's saying in response to minor moments that "I am not cut out for this." "I am a bad mom." "I can't do anything right." "I am not maternal." "Breastfeeding is supposed to be natural." "Everyone else does it better than me." "Something is wrong with me because it's not working." It's attaching a mistake to your being and letting it define you. Most importantly, it's a distortion.

The difference between mom guilt and mom shame is that mom guilt is "I did something bad," and mom shame is "I am bad." In cognitive behavioral therapy, we call the thoughts that attach to these feelings of guilt and shame cognitive distortions. When we are feeling overwhelmed, stressed, sick, depressed, or anxious, we tend to think more distorted thoughts. That's because it's easier to think bad thoughts when you feel bad. We can also be more vulnerable to distorted thoughts when we feel insecure, like when we have our first baby and everything is new. Or when we have our second baby and it's different and everything is still new, but you think, *I should know this already.*

To reiterate, the frequency, severity, and depths of mom shame should be viewed as symptoms. You may be prone to mom shame because you're a perfectionist, had a critical parent, suffered from past trauma, or because you're in the thick of a really tough moment or development stage. If it's happening often, lasts long, and is severe, ask yourself if you are depressed, anxious, or overwhelmed? Is this reflective of an unresolved trauma coming up? Do you need more support from a partner or need to fill your soul with a creative and meaningful activity? Do you need more help, such as a well-trained therapist, to help you sort through the shame you are experiencing? When motherhood throws you to the wolves, the wolf you feed will win.

When working with patients, I teach them about all different types of cognitive distortions, including black-and-white thinking (e.g., "I am failing at motherhood"), mind reading (thinking that other mothers know exactly what they're doing), "should" statements (e.g., "I should know how to do this"), catastrophic thinking (the worst-case scenario will happen), and magnification and minimization (exaggerating a small detail's importance and minimizing the positive). These patterns can be broken. The first step is to help my patients recognize the distortions and generally understand when their thinking is faulty. After they identify that they are having a distorted thought, I encourage them to challenge the thought and come up with a more rational, well-rounded, open-minded thought. Typically, I have them practice working through the thought on paper or a chart to come up with more rational thoughts. By seeing it in front of them, they can understand just how distorted the thought actually is and then come up with a more well-rounded thought.

Try this related exercise: imagine the irrational worry or thought is being presented in a court of law. Brainstorm the actual facts that support the irrational thought and the facts that go against the thought. Then you can look through the evidence—and hint: usually there are almost no actual facts supporting the irrational worry. Then you come up with a more balanced, well-rounded thought.

Let's run through an example. A patient of mine, Cara, reported that she was feeling dejected because she thought her baby's pediatrician thought she was a "bad mother." When I asked why she thought that, she explained that she brought her eight-month-old to the doctor and admitted that she had not introduced a "variety of solid foods" into her baby's diet. The pediatrician told her to feed the baby at least three "meals" and two snacks on top of 25 to 32 ounces of formula. My patient was overwhelmed at the thought of introducing solids on top of everything else, and making time for five additional feedings felt impossible to her.

As a result, Cara thought, *I am a bad mother.* This cognitive distortion is an example of black-and-white or all-or-nothing thinking. Cara, like a lot of mothers, was feeling overwhelmed, stressed, and anxious, which was further preventing her from introducing new foods. When working with Cara, first it was important to soften her shame. I encouraged her to speak to herself the way she would speak to a friend, with kindness and compassion. In addition, it was important that she acknowledge that anxiety was the main barrier to getting her to introduce solids, as it is for so many new moms. It is not her fault that she has anxiety, and now that she is in treatment, we can work toward better supporting her through this important developmental phase for her baby.

Soften on Mom Shame

- Shame is taking those momentary blips and making them signals when they are just noise.
- Think about the way you are thinking. In cognitive behavioral therapy we view thoughts, feelings, and behaviors as interrelated and influencing each other. There are cognitive, emotion-focused, and behavioral strategies that can improve our functioning.
- Cognitive distortions are thought errors. The most common types of distortions are:
- Black-and-white/all-or-nothing thinking: rigid, extreme thinking (e.g., *I am failing at motherhood*).
- Mind reading: thinking that you know what another person is thinking (e.g., *These other mothers know exactly what they are doing*).
- Should statements: any statement with "should" in it (e.g., *I should know how to do this*). Remove the word "should" from your vocabulary.
- Catastrophizing: thinking the worst possible outcome will happen (e.g., *If I don't breastfeed my baby, they will have something wrong with them and it will be my fault*).
- Magnification and minimization: exaggerating a small detail's importance and minimizing the positive (e.g., *I forgot to fill out the doctor's form for daycare. I keep forgetting. I am so stupid and can't remember* anything).
- We are more likely to think distorted thoughts when we are depressed, anxious, or feeling bad physically.

One of the main responsibilities of a parent in the first year is to feed your baby. There is something so rewarding about a baby with thigh rolls and chubby cheeks. It is satisfying when a baby takes in what you give them. Congratulations if your six-month-old eats asparagus and foie gras. For many moms, though, worries about allergies and choking hazards come up.

I asked Cara to imagine her pediatrician was actually accusing her of being a bad mother. What was the factual evidence? She paused.

Mind reading falls under cognitive distortion as well. What evidence do you have that your pediatrician thinks you are a bad mother? Did she say that to you?

Can you think of specific examples that you are a good mother? There are so many things we do for our babies minute to minute. Some examples include scheduling and attending important medical appointments, regularly feeding your baby, and soothing, dressing, playing with, and providing physical affection for your baby. A more rational, well-rounded thought for this patient would be: I am nervous about introducing a variety of solid foods to my baby, and I have a plan in place to do so. I am getting treatment for my anxiety. I am working on this transition. Transitions are difficult and they take time.

Now, if I look at this through my diagnostic clinical lens, I see the anxiety and avoidance cycle. While a plan is in place, anxiety is playing a role. I did work with this patient in completing anxiety treatment exposure exercises for introducing solids. We even worked on getting her partner involved to do the feedings because that counts too.

Over time, the patient and her husband would introduce more varieties of foods, including puréed nuts, eggs, grains, fruits, and vegetables. She was anxious about nut allergies due to family history, so she had her baby tested for allergies and conducted the first nut exposures in the allergist's office. Then they were conducted in the parking lot of the local emergency room. Then at home.

Gradually, Cara became less anxious about introducing foods and gave herself some compassion. She was able to more clearly see how she focused too much on her own shame. She is more able to see how she is a good mother for lots of reasons, even when she feels that she is falling behind in one task. I encouraged her to stop comparing herself to others and to challenge her automatic cognitive distortions when they come up. Of note: by doing exposures and treating her anxiety, she was also able to think in more well-rounded and rational ways.

When we are in an anxious state, it's hard to problem-solve. So it's also important to take deep breaths, practice mindfulness, and slow things down. It is not an emergency, even though it may feel like it is. Try to calm your body down first, and then you will be better able to think more clearly.

With mom shame, check in with that inner child being criticized, the one who could use some mothering, some compassion, and some tenderness. Another strategy I recommend is to write a letter to yourself in the way you would write to a mom friend. I recommend giving yourself very specific feedback about all the things that went well that day. There are so many things! We do a thousand things a day. If three do not go as we expected, that's still nearly 100 percent. If 30 things go wrong, it's 97 percent. If 300 things go wrong, we're still winning the majority.

Here's an example of a letter I would write to myself.

Dear Me,

You did a great job with the baby today. When he cried when he did not want to take a nap, you held him. You soothed him. You then played peekaboo through the crib and read him a book before leaving the room. Before you dropped him off at daycare, you puréed some butternut squash and peas for his snacks and remembered to bring the refill container of rice cereal. Great job getting some vegetables in there. You could have easily tossed in the applesauce pouch and baby yogurt like yesterday. But you did it differently today because Mike gave you some extra time to sleep in and you had more in your tank.

As you write this, I know you are still focusing on that extra screen time you used with Jordan after you got Max to sleep. I know you feel guilty, and I wonder if that mommy message of perfectionism is coming up again, as it seems to be slightly torturing you. That screen time allowed you to take a hot shower that you so desperately needed. That seems to have triggered that recurrent neural pathway in your brain, the pathway that lights up every time the old message that you *have to be perfect to be a good mom* is triggered. Every time you focus on compassion for yourself, instead of giving in to the perfectionism, you are working to break down that old neural network. You are working so hard to build new roads in your brain, new paths of the motherhood journey. The more you can let that go, the more new highways will emerge. That old wound of perfectionism will be lost. Keep up the great work. You are a fighter. Try to shift your mindset to something else that went well today, like washing Jordan's hair with shampoo and her body with soap, putting conditioner in her hair, and brushing out the knots in her hair in the shower; or how you did Max's laundry so that he would have a clean swaddle for bedtime; or how you bathed and fed them while Mike had to work late. These are just a couple of examples of what you did for your little ones today. I know there is so much more.

Love, Me

In treatment, I provide therapy that works to build new neural networks. Therapy can rewire your brain. Here, I work to rewire the brain on motherhood. The more we can reinforce new, protective, compassionate, self-fulfilled, and healing roads, the more we can let the forest grow over those old roads that may have been instilled from our own wounded mothers, our perfectionism, our trying to adhere to the idealistic image of the selfless mother. The good news is that there will be millions of opportunities to keep checking in with yourself and identify the guilt and the shame. Those terrible feelings are opportunities to choose a different road. Every time you do, you are mothering yourself and breaking the cycle.

Just as I offered with maternal guilt, here are some common mom shame statements and their healthy reframe statements. However, shame statements tend to be bigger, core beliefs. They are almost always cognitive distortions because they are extreme statements. While reframing can be helpful, other strategies are needed because shame represents beliefs about yourself, likely deep wounds. It is also helpful to recognize the pain you are suffering, acknowledge how hard you are being on yourself, and demonstrate self-compassion to that inner child who is feeling shame.

Mom Shame Says: *I am not a good mother.*
Healthy Reframe: No one is all good or all bad. This is an example of the black-and-white thinking cognitive distortion. There are parts of each of us that can benefit from practice, patience, and further development. I don't have to be perfect to be good.

Mom Shame Says: *I don't have maternal instinct. Something is wrong with me.*
Healthy Reframe: Maternal instinct is a myth. There are some things that you rely on instinct for, and you did that with _____. More commonly, it's trial and error and practice over time.

Mom Shame Says: *Everyone else knows how to do this better than me. I am a failure.*
Healthy Reframe: We rarely see the full picture. I am drawing con-clusions from limited information (cognitive distortion). Motherhood is challenging for most. It's important for me to validate my authentic experience and take care of myself.

Mom Shame Says: *I am lacking something "motherly."*
Healthy Reframe: Challenge this distortion in a court of law. Be spe-cific. It was motherly when I soothed my baby today. It was motherly when I held my baby and prepared the bottle. I was motherly when I exercised and tended to my own needs so that I could be a more present mother for my baby.

Mom Shame Says: *Breastfeeding is supposed to be natural.*
Healthy Reframe: Sometimes breastfeeding is easy. Oftentimes, there are challenges based on circumstances out of our control. What is most natural is wanting to feed and nourish your baby. Try to be flexible and problem-solve if challenges come up. It's okay to feel disappointed/relieved/thrilled/angry if breastfeeding does not work.

Mom Shame Says: *Something is wrong with me because I don't love this time with my new baby.*
Healthy Reframe: Ambivalence is the norm in early motherhood.

Remember, mom shame is any statement or feeling that represents "I am bad." It is a core distortion and will not serve you in motherhood. Work on challenging those beliefs with more well-rounded, compas-sionate thoughts. Imagine you are speaking to a friend when you talk to yourself. Would you ever say those statements to a friend? No. So why would you say that to yourself? Be kind to yourself.

Soften on Mom Shame

- When you experience mom shame, try imagining you are in a court of law and only present the facts that support and refute the thought (cognitive distortion) associated with the shame. Come up with a healthy and more rational reframe.
- Slow things down and tend to your needs. When we are feeling anxious, it is difficult to problem-solve and think clearly.
- Ask yourself: Is your inner child feeling criticized? How can you nurture your inner child and break the cycle? Use compassion and tenderness. Try writing yourself a letter like you would to a mom friend, commenting on what went well that day. Be as specific as possible. As primary caregivers, we do a million things per day.
- Therapy changes your brain. It helps you build stronger and more positive neural networks. It rewires the faulty system. I tell my patients we are building new highways. We have to clear the path and continuously choose to reinforce those paths. We have to let trees grow over those old negative neural networks by taking different roads. Over time, those maladaptive neural paths will be lost.

I click on "Admit Patient" on the telehealth meeting to let Marissa into our session. As soon as she sees me appear on screen, she starts. "I had lunch with my close friend this week. You know, the one I told you about who has been reading a million parenting books. Anyway, she always seems to know what she is doing. I feel like a terrible mother. I had this special day planned with my baby where we were going to go to a mommy-and-me yoga class. I had planned a meetup with other local moms I have been trying to connect with for some time. I was already running late, and Kayla fell asleep in the car on the way there. When I went to take her into the class she just cried the whole time. I tried to calm her down in the hallway, but after about 10 minutes I gave up and went home. I feel like a failure."

I listen intently and settle into my chair.

"Can you tell me what you did before the class?" I asked. "Start from when you woke up."

"Sure, so I woke up around 5:30 AM," Marissa recalled. "Kayla was hungry. I gave her a bottle. I burped her, changed her, and then got her dressed in this cute little onesie I have been waiting for her to grow into. I was excited to take her out and show her off. You should have seen her—it was a pale pink with tulle that looked like a ballerina skirt. The footies had ballet slippers etched in with bright pink thread. I never thought I would love pink so much until I had a girl. After I got her dressed, I had to keep her awake until her next naptime at 10 AM. I am trying to get her on this new schedule that may be a little easier for when I have both the baby and her sister home. I took her downstairs and read her some books. Then she did some tummy time. I puréed her food for the day while she rocked in the baby swing. It was only 7:30 by then. The mommy-and-me class was at 9 AM, so I took her for a walk in the stroller to the playground and pushed her in the baby swing for a little bit. Then I gave her another bottle at the park and burped her. I changed her diaper when we got home, then headed out the door for mommy-and-me. I tried to get all the things done before the class so she wouldn't be hungry or uncomfortable. Then she fell asleep and all was lost."

"So let me see if I understand what you are telling me," I said. "You spent essentially half of a typical workday, about four hours, tending to all her needs and making sure she was fed, comfortable, entertained, and amused, and then because she fell asleep you failed?" I try to exaggerate the cognitive distortion for her.

"Yeah, but I really wanted this plan to work out and meet the other mommies," Marissa lamented. "How do they always get there on time?

How do they always get everything together—one mommy even had a matching yoga outfit with her baby! I saw them through the door. The mommies were doing these cute little downward dogs, cooing and giggling with their babies below them. I'll never be like that."

"Hmmm," I nod. "Where do think this feeling of not ever being good enough comes from?"

"Probably from my overcritical dad. He told me I was never good enough. I am sure it comes from him. But I don't want to get into that. I need practical advice, like what do I do when I am so upset because my baby won't stick to the napping schedule, or wakes up in the middle of the night, or has a blowout right after I bathe her and I have to do it all over again," she said tearfully.

"I understand. So in these moments that push you over the edge, you feel triggered and lash out," I said. "What you really need to do is slow things down and fill your cup. The problem is not that the baby is doing all these things you mention—although annoying, they are developmentally appropriate. Although you don't see it when you look through the mommy-and-me yoga class, those moms are dealing with most of the same struggles," I said, trying to reassure her. "You feel that you are doing something wrong when these things happen, and it reminds you of your critical father,"

I then explained further. "When you start thinking these distorted thoughts and feel triggered, your body responds as if you are in danger, but you are not. There are two questions I always want you to ask yourself when you feel triggered: 1) Is this an emergency? and 2) Is my baby going to die? If those two answers are no, you can take a moment. Listen for the most distant sound you can hear. Practice mindfulness. Take a beat. Breathe and soften. Ask yourself how can you be kinder to yourself in this moment?"

"I have a really hard time not jumping up and taking care of Kayla when she cries. I have a visceral reaction in my body. It physically hurts to hear her cry," she said.

"A lot of moms experience that reaction," I explained. "It's okay to pause and slow things down. Your brain and body will want to respond to the baby quickly, but it's equally important that you tend to your needs as well. Perhaps you try to pause for a minute before you grab her and see if you can get some deep belly breaths in, or pee, or maybe drink some water before you start the routine."

"And listen to her cry?" she jumped in.

"Yes, for a minute. Or even 30 seconds. Practice checking in with yourself and it will become easier over time," I said.

Psychologist Donald Winnicott coined the term "good enough mother," referring to the gradual increases of slight frustration that occur from birth on. For example, at first the mother attends to every single one of the newborn's needs. As the baby matures, more gradual intervals of time are introduced between meeting the needs. A mother may wait a couple of minutes before responding to her three-month-old's cries. This is a natural process of development, and the space between getting the need met by the mother allows the baby to differentiate between their internal and external worlds. Plus, the world is not perfect, so by being a "good enough mother," you are modeling imperfections in life and in relationships. I remind my patients like Marissa that we live in a perfectionist culture that can be toxic. Mothers are striving to be perfect, and it's not healthy for anyone. "Good enough mothering" is enough, and in these spaces we can use them to our advantage. Between the moments of caring for and tending to our babies needs we can infuse some activities, self-care, therapy, and replenishing for ourselves, reminding ourselves how essential our needs are as well.

Brené Brown speaks of an excellent strategy for not instilling shame in her children and even her dog. When her dog or kids make a mistake or do something wrong, she says, "Bad choice," not "Bad dog" or "Bad boy." Everyone can make a bad choice or a mistake, especially ourselves when we are stressed, depressed, sleep-deprived, anxious, overwhelmed, developing, and learning in this new mothering role. I take Brown's strategy one step further. To soften on mom shame, if you make a questionable choice or a mistake, say "Bad choice" to yourself and follow up with, "I am still learning. I will make a better choice the next time because this experience has given me more information that can help me." If you change the statements to "bad choice" or "make a better choice next time" instead of "you're a bad mother," it takes shame out of the equation. Remember, shame is "I am bad." It's never too late to speak to yourself in a compassionate way.

SNAPSHOT

Soften on Mom Shame

- When you are feeling triggered, ask yourself two questions:
  - Is this an emergency?
  - Is my baby going to die?
- If both answers are no, tend to your own needs first.
- Be mindful if you are being overly critical or punitive. Try not to get stuck on "Why me?" but ask yourself, "What now?"
- Slow down. Check in and take your "temperature." What do you need?
- When we are present and less stressed, we can have better access to all our psychological resources—our superpowers.
- Even further, if you can get yourself into a playful, positive mood and an uplifted state, you will have even greater access to your maternal psychological resources. This is because a positive mood leads to a more open mind, greater creativity, and more cognitive flexibility, all of which are integral to thriving in motherhood.

9

EMBRACE YOUR NEW MOM RAGE

"Be prepared to dance with your feelings." (on mom rage)
—ANNE LAMOTT, WRITER AND MOTHER OF ONE, *OPERATING INSTRUCTIONS*

"Will you please eat that rice cereal faster," I thought as I smiled tensely at my baby grinning and playing with his baby slop with his fingers on his high chair tray. I tried so hard to keep grinning at him and cooing while I kept feeding him. I tried not to scream, but I could feel my chest getting tight. The clock read 8:19 PM, and the bath time, changing, swaddling, and rocking multistep bedtime routine still loomed. I had a particularly inspiring session that day with a patient, and I knew I had to get my thoughts on paper as soon as possible or I might lose some of the details. I repeated the highlights in my mind while glaring at the clock. Unbeknownst to my husband, the pinball had been launched and left rattling around in my body. The mom rage was triggered.

Mom rage is an all-or-nothing phenomenon. I could feel the anger pulse through my veins as my husband walked down the stairs. He had just completed a workout on the bike, and I snapped at him. I made some snide remark suggesting that it must be nice to get exercise in and can you read my mind and take care of our baby now?! I knew full well that we had a division of labor, a verbal allocation of tasks. He did the bath time routine with Max and the bedtime with Jordan, and I did the bath with Jordan and bedtime with Max. "What's up with you?" he asked.

"I really need to write this passage for my book, and it's taking a long time for Max to eat this cereal. I'm trying to see if it will help his belly be more full so he doesn't wake up in the middle of the night. It seems like he's going through a growth spurt. It's been really rough with the frequent wakings. Even though you get him, I still wake up because I can hear him cry. It's hard for me to get back to sleep."

"Well, lucky for you your actual job is not writing that book."

I paused. I eyed the kitchen counter and thought I had better stay away from any sharp objects. Scratch that—sharp or dull objects, because in that moment I could have killed him with the baby spoon in my hand. I handed the spoon to Max to let him play with it just in case I were to lose control of my body. I am convinced that there is a biologically protective reason why my mom rage was targeted at my husband and not my baby, and for that I am grateful. It is much safer to want to kill your husband.

Many things happened in that moment. The mom rage was at an all-time, overboiled, teakettle-screaming-on-the-stove high. There was no turning back. There is no antidote for mom rage in the moment. The only thing you can do is not make things worse. That's it. In the moment, once it is released in your body, only a horse tranquilizer could settle that feeling. You are trapped by the intense rage and most likely fear its force, not knowing where it will land.

I repeated to myself: the best I can do is not make it worse. Don't make it worse. What this means is don't take the bait. I could have easily gotten into it with my husband, telling him that he is not a writer. That he doesn't understand what happens in your soul when you have the next chapter on hand. The need to get it out on paper for fear it could be lost forever. I could have easily gone into a rant about how I always do bedtime with Max and expressed resentment. I could have even taken the rice cereal away from Max to go to bed faster, but then he might not sleep through the night, and I couldn't risk that either. I could have easily asked my husband to take over, but he would have likely pushed back. He had just been on call for the past week, and we have spoken often about how he needs time to take care of himself too—especially after being available 24/7 for days on end and tending to patient emergencies. Having another conversation about that in that moment would have just prolonged the delay in getting back to my writing. I could have done all this and given in to my rage. That would have undoubtedly made things worse. It would have increased the tension with my husband. It would have increased the likelihood of me being sleep-deprived and more irritable as a result. None of these responses would have helped me in the moment.

Don't get me wrong, I still wanted to throttle my husband. Honestly, the intensity of mom rage could have carried me through that task, I am sure of it. Even in my rage, I was able to have a few rational thoughts: we had agreed to this division of responsibility, he is taking care of himself, and if it is not working for me I can make a point to discuss this with him when I have my wits about me. I could have focused on his response, amplifying that he could have been more sensitive, more empathic, more helpful to me. However, it was an off moment and he was not reading the volcanic lava bubbling up below my skin. The moment was incongruent to the man who stayed up reading my book, chapter by chapter, and laughed, encouraging me to write more. This moment was incongruent to the partner who generously offered up permission to include our personal stories from our marriage and family life, which we both consider sacred.

But that mom rage. It's a truly terrible feeling wrapped in hormones, fatigue, unmet needs, and the competing demands of life and babies in such a dependent stage. The babies are need machines just taking, taking, and taking. I am not saying you will have the wherewithal to immediately see things clearly in a mom rage state; you likely won't. I was able to have a glimpse of rational thought because I do this for a living and focus on meeting so many of my needs. With practice and by slowing the rage down, we can all get there.

In the meantime, it will take all your strength during moments of mom rage, and I mean all of it, *not to make things worse*. It took every single ounce of my being to stay silent toward my husband, to move through the bedtime routine with Max as a path of least resistance. Once he was down, I marched into the bedroom, clinging to my only goal of getting that chapter out, and snatched my computer from my nightstand. En route, I passed my husband, lying feet up, watching a documentary about wildebeests. I thought sarcastically, *How relaxing for you, Honey*. But again, I ignored the bait, knowing that would have only delayed me from getting where I needed to be. I quickly walked downstairs, shut the door to my office, and wrote for two hours. After the two hours were up, the mom rage passed and my husband was still alive.

SNAPSHOT

Embrace Your New Mom Rage

- The most important rule with mom rage is: do not make things worse.
- Don't take the bait into power struggles or fight with your partner.
- Mom rage is an all-or-nothing phenomenon. Once the trigger is released, it has to run its course. Hold steady. I repeat, *do not make things worse*.
- Mom rage is fueled by hormones, lack of sleep, feeling depleted, not having needs met, and being pulled in too many directions. Yes, there are absolutely societal contributors, but let's focus on what we can control in the moment and in the meantime until things change.
- Don't try to figure out your trigger in the moment.
- Focus on the quickest route to get you to getting your needs met. Beware the landmines.

Mom rage is very common. If you are anything like me, you may not have experienced the depths of rage until you became a mother. Until you were depleted. Until you were sleep-deprived and being pulled in too many directions—mom, wife, sister, friend, colleague, employee, owner, homemaker, and others—all in the same day and sometimes in the same minute. Until the relentlessness sunk in. Until the too many competing needs went to war. Until you danced with the depths of something dark.

Just this morning, my husband offered to take Max to daycare and Jordan to school. I eagerly anticipated drinking hot coffee in bed while rewatching the latest episode of *Succession* that I didn't make it through the previous night. The day prior, in a moment of feeling uncharacteristically motivated, I had meal-prepped some puréed fruits and vegetables for the week, feeling like I too could be a Pinterest mom. I labeled the containers with the days of the week so we could easily grab them in the morning on the way to daycare. I was feeling prepared to take on the week, knowing full well that this would probably be the first and last week of baby meal prep. But, hey, I could snap a picture and save it in my photos as proof that I did in fact give my baby fresh food in case anybody asked. And I could convince myself for a brief minute that no, I don't "desperately need" those best-things-ever-invented gifts from heaven: premade baby pouches.

I settled into my pillows and began drinking my hot coffee, only to be interrupted by a phone call from my husband saying that he forgot Max's purées in the fridge. In my head, I was raging, *How on earth could you forget the purées? I reminded you this morning to grab them from the fridge. The day was labeled. How could I make this any easier for you?!* I did not say this out loud, of course. Because saying those things would not turn back time and make the purées magically appear at daycare today. It would only make my husband feel worse and not want to help out again.

I stuffed that rage deep down and took a breath. "Can you drop them off at daycare? Oh, and they're running low on his diaper cream. Can you grab that too?" he asked, to which I responded, "Yes, it's fine."

I wasn't thrilled. He knew that. He even said, "What am I, stupid? Is that what you want to say?" As if he read my mind. If I reacted and said those types of insults, that would only make this annoying scenario worse. Plus, it's helpful to not dwell on that thing because the next thing is coming up any minute. You both need your resources to handle the next curveball. Trust me, with new babies and littles, it's coming. I looked down at my coffee and said, "No, no. It happens." I finished the cup, then dropped the purées off for Max. The world kept turning.

Experiencing mom rage does not mean you are dark. It also does not mean you are a bad mother. I assess mom rage similar to mom guilt and mom shame: as a symptom. Are you tired, depleted, bored, angry, depressed, anxious, triggered, and overworked? Do you need a break? Do you need to have a proactive conversation or many conversations with your partner to discuss the breakdown of responsibilities? Are you disappointed? Is this not what you expected and are you having a difficult time adjusting?

One of my patients, Melany, sought therapy for her "temper," stating that she never used to be a yeller, but that she has been so angry lately and can't help it. Her husband prompted her to see someone. Melany had opted not to go back to work after her first baby. She decided to be a stay-at-home mother and confided that she always wanted to do that because she was raised in a home where one parent worked the night shift and the other the day shift. She recalled always wanting more time with her parents when she was young.

At first, she liked having the time with her baby and being so hands-on. She enjoyed the walks to the park, the feedings, the cuddles, and bath time. But the baby was now 11 months old, and her feelings were not the same. Her enjoyment of these experiences was starting to dwindle.

Melany explained that the baby had started walking, so she had to constantly monitor her for safety and also felt the pressure to keep her stimulated during the day. She admitted that she was not enjoying this phase as much as the early days of infancy. Melany also didn't tell her husband because she didn't want him to think she was a bad mother. She didn't tell her close friends because they all seemed to love being stay-at-home mothers. She thought something was wrong with her. She thought she wasn't cut out for this.

At night, she and her husband would have dinner and then spend time together with the baby. She did take time for herself to shower and listen to a podcast while she folded laundry. However, she rarely went out with her friends because she was tired. They had not looked for a babysitter yet because her mother-in-law watched the baby when they needed someone. She and her husband went out to dinner occasionally. She didn't mind because she was focused on the baby. However, she found herself feeling irritable and snapping at her husband.

"Did you not think to dry the floor? Do I have to tell you every single thing? Use your brain!" Melany recounted saying to him. She lamented, "I don't understand. It's like he doesn't think of these things that are so obvious. Like the other day, he said he went to the other room to get his phone, left her 'for a second,' he says, and of course he returned to find her crying and covered with books after she had pulled them off the shelves. He left her in the living room, where she was playing with her stuffies, and the next minute she was in trouble. I have explained to him countless times that he can't take his eyes off her when he is watching her. That things happen in a split second. That he has to anticipate potential hazards. It's like I can't get a break. It bothers me that he doesn't seem to take it seriously."

This example may seem simple, but upon further examination, so many common themes are occurring. First, Melany is the primary caregiver, which means she's psychologically responsible for the baby. It's difficult, if not impossible, to shut that off. It is a responsibility and a weight like no other. No one tells you about the complete hijacking of your psyche that occurs with a baby. Especially in the early years of parenting, when young ones are so dependent, so many psychological and physical resources from the primary caregiver are needed to tend to the children's needs. In this case, Melany and her husband psychologically negotiated these roles, and the father/husband is simply not oriented in this way. That is a thing, but it's not a bad thing. They also negotiated this trade-off before they became parents, before she became a mother.

Second, Melany is depleted. She is exhausted. She is critical of herself for not "enjoying" this phase of motherhood as she thought she would and as she set out to do. She is internalizing the challenges as faults in herself. She thinks she is failing.

Third, she is anxious. Yes, a certain hypervigilance is required in motherhood to keep your baby safe. And Melany is doing a great job keeping her baby safe. However, she is also avoiding leaving the baby, not allowing others to step in and help, and is rigid in her thinking. She assumes that any injuries, boo-boos, or lapses in hyperattunement to the baby are negative, dangerous, and should never occur. Yes, we want to prevent danger, and no, we cannot prevent every mishap. The husband will benefit from more parenting experience. The patient will benefit from some relief from the relentless responsibilities of motherhood.

In working with Melany, I helped her, like so many of my patients, in the following ways. I encouraged her to approach motherhood and her transition to being a mother with curiosity instead of criticism. She has never been a mother to an 11-month-old baby, so how on earth would she know how she felt about it before she did it? She is learning that she does not care for this particular phase as much as infancy, and that is okay. She may come to find out that she likes the next phase more, or not at all, but she loves adolescence—who knows? You don't have to love every phase, every minute, every holiday, every night of parenthood to be a good mother. I encourage my patients to explore, notice, accept and validate their feelings—they are all okay. Once we know what we are feeling, we can problem-solve.

Problem-solving with this patient looked like enrolling the baby in a daycare program a couple of days a week; hiring a babysitter for one night a week so Melany could have time with her husband; and encouraging her to explore new hobbies, creative ventures, or part-time work options. In addition, anxiety treatment was provided. Cognitive distortions around motherhood and her spouse were challenged to help her think more flexibly. She was encouraged to leave her baby with others more often for exposure treatment. This would purposefully make her more anxious at first, and then, over time, she would become more comfortable, could leave for longer periods of time, and could focus on other things. She began to reap the benefits of socializing more, engaging in creative activities, exercising, and filling her cup. This allowed her to also think more flexibly, be less reactive, and thwart mom rage episodes. She was able to slow things down, take notice, and observe herself in nonjudgmental ways.

Beyond the practical strategies, time was spent grieving the childhood Melany did not have and the parental closeness she craved. It is important for her to acknowledge this loss and let it rest. In many ways she is breaking the cycle and spending more time with her daughter, but she went to the other extreme, which was not working for her. When we are consumed by rage, anxiety, and depression, we are also not emotionally available to tend to our babies as well. So, in another way, if Melany continued down the path she was on, she was at risk for repeating a version of the same trauma. Emily Oster, PhD, economist and author of Cribsheet, spoke about the quality, not quantity, of hours with her children. She noticed that her quality of being present with her littles started to diminish when she spent more than three hours at a time with them. I tend to tap out around four hours on average. However, sometimes, if I am on empty, I can tap out at 15 minutes.

I also worked with Melany to identify her specific triggers. This is important because identifying themes or repeated triggers can help predict when you are vulnerable and more likely to be triggered. This allows you to put on your armor before the situation at hand, and it also allows you to notice when you are triggered more quickly so you can respond. For my patient, her triggers seemed to be around her baby potentially getting physically injured. No one wants their baby to get hurt. But it's one thing to be upset about it or try to protect your baby. It's another thing to be triggered. It's important to know the difference in how it feels and how it makes you think. When we have an extreme reaction, it is likely that personal history is contributing to the dynamic. In other words, this trigger had deep roots for my patient because she broke her leg in a car accident as an adolescent, had to have a metal rod inserted in her leg, and missed out on an important season of varsity track. She never fully recovered and had to forfeit her early running career. It's also important to know that not all triggers come from a major life experience. They can come from big and small experiences. Neither makes them any more valid than the other.

Melany experienced episodes of mom rage less when she started taking care of herself more. She still had some triggering episodes of mom rage because, well, it is still motherhood. There are still too many competing needs. However, she was able to accept her feelings and respond productively instead of displacing them in destructive ways (e.g., internal criticism or yelling at her husband). She became more forgiving of herself and more compassionate. Her self-talk changed from "You aren't cut out for this," to "This is a hard moment in motherhood; let's see how we can shift things." By protecting her brain from starting a negative spiral, she could think more openly. When we feel really bad, we tend to think more narrow, rigid thoughts. It's important to notice when you are triggered, but try to refrain from focusing on "Why am I triggered?" and instead move into the more important question, "What now?" If we can help ourselves feel better, even just a little bit better, our mind opens and we can think more clearly. Then, when we are calm, we can think about the episode and what was going on underneath. A skilled therapist can also help you sort that out. Motherhood can be a relentless series of problem-solving.

As a side note, when I searched through PubMed for the scholarly research articles and studies investigating maternal rage, I was surprised to find "0" next to the results. Some studies had nothing to do with motherhood, and a bunch of rodent studies investigating something with the acronym RAGE had nothing to do with actual maternal rage. *This can't be correct*, I thought. I retyped "mom rage" and was met with similar results. It was perplexing, given that there are no shortage of reports from my patients, mom friends, and the media about this phenomenon. Mom rage was quite literally all the rage, and accounts of triggers included being touched out by babies and toddlers, a partner asking them to do one more thing, another mess, another boo-boo, temper tantrums, unfair division of labor, unmet needs, another sick day, and another incident that invokes the feeling of not being in control. I thought about my search some more.

I entered "maternal anger" in the search box. Low and behold, research articles appeared in the context of postpartum depression. When we think about the difference between rage and anger, we can think of them along a continuum. However, they are very different experiences. Anger is less intense. Rage is very intense, can be destructive, and can also be violent.

When mothers experience mom rage, it is nearly intolerable. Many of my patients say that the intensity of the anger is something they have not experienced before the throes of motherhood. Many moms feel ashamed or guilty when their rage takes over. Remember to be kind to yourself. It is better not to have an emotion on top of an emotion. Observe your rage, but don't complicate it further by adding shame and guilt. Allow the rage to run its course through your veins and validate that you are having a tough emotional experience.

My conversations with my patients about their experience around mom rage is to ask their triggers, frequency of episodes, severity/intensity of episodes, and duration of episodes.

Maternal rage can be a warning sign that your tank is on empty and needs to be refueled, now. It's important to understand your specific maternal rage triggers. By understanding repetitive patterns, you can identify what is driving the rage underneath. The triggers can stem from seemingly simpler things like lack of sleep and unmet daily needs, to more complex losses, childhood trauma, and dynamics with your parents from childhood. But the middle of a mom rage episode is not time to explore the "why." In the moment, lean in to the strategies.

SNAPSHOT

Embrace Your New Mom Rage

- Many mothers have not experienced the depths of rage until they became a mother. Experiencing mom rage does not mean you are dark, bad, or wrong.
- Ask yourself, are you tired? Depleted? Angry? Depressed? Anxious? Triggered? Overworked?
- Can you problem-solve around this? Have conversations with your partner to discuss roles and responsibilities. Discuss division of labor at a time when you are not feeling rageful.
- Do you need more help? More time to yourself?
- Mom rage can be a symptom of underlying depression and anxiety. Consult with a mental health provider for an objective assessment if you are experiencing mom rage. A provider can help you understand your mom rage and provide treatment and coping skills.
- Be open to renegotiating roles and responsibilities with your partner throughout parenthood. Some things you signed up for might not work in every phase of development or stage of life. Have many check-in conversations to renegotiate if needed.
- Many mothers experience shame and guilt when they feel mom rage. Try to just have a "clean" mom rage feeling without a complicated feeling (e.g., shame or guilt) on top. It is healthier to just allow yourself to have the feeling. This is also a strategy to not make the mom rage worse.
- The antidote to mom rage is becoming lighter in that moment. Slow down. Contain. Breathe. Steady yourself. Do less.

10

HOW TO MANAGE A MATERNAL MENTAL HEALTH CRISIS

*"Proclaimed the time was neither wrong nor right, I have
been one acquainted with the night."*
—ROBERT FROST, "ACQUAINTED WITH THE NIGHT"

After having my first child, managing postpartum anxiety, and moving through the identity transition of becoming a mother, I was ready to do it all over again! *This time*, I thought, *I would be prepared.* I had already become a mother, so I wouldn't have to go through *that* identity transformation again. It would be, quite literally, more of the same. Even though I was 30 to 70 percent more likely to get postpartum OCD again because I had it once before, although a much milder version, I did not think that I would get it again because I had mastered the treatment. I had this in the bag.

You can imagine my utter shock when my once again perfectly intact ego was completely shattered from the return of postpartum OCD with a vengeance, and none of the strategies that had worked for me previously worked any longer. The octopus death spiral felt too close for comfort.

After Max was born, I had minimal physical pain, and my plan to return to normalcy felt like it was on track. In fact, I felt so good that I quickly dismissed the routine social worker mental health visit. My nurses were pleasantly surprised when they found me walking laps around the unit just one day after my C-section. I bounced around the hospital, visiting my son in the Neonatal Intensive Care Unit (NICU) and then heading back to my room every chance I got.

When I returned home, I slipped into my jeans and was thrilled that I could practically close the top button with some minor acrobatics. Looking in the mirror, almost wearing my non-mom jeans, I caught a glimpse of my black belted blazer, one of my go-to presentation outfits. I was eager to wear that blazer again, tie that belt around my soon-to-be-cinched waist, and get right back into my flourishing private practice. Like a train heading down a track at full speed, I had simply gotten off at an early stop and taken a small journey with Max, but I would catch up later down the track and jump back on, ready to drive and without losing speed. After nine long months of hyperemesis, I could feel the essence of me coming through, ready to burst at a moment's notice. I missed the rigors and productivity of academia, a full social life, and date nights with my husband. We had gotten back into taking vacations together and regularly scheduled concerts before I got pregnant again. It seemed like everything was on pause until now, and I had my finger on the play button, ready to press.

After Jordan was born, I had taken five months off work and barely wore anything but oversized T-shirts and leggings. I would lie on the couch for hours with her, cuddling, reading, with the occasional venture outside to a mommy-and-me class or walk around town. I was oriented to her every need and forgot about my own. Jordan was the only thing to see, and for sure, the only thing I saw. This time, I would regain a sense of myself sooner. This was the mother I wanted to be, closer to who I was before giving birth: adventurous, well versed in the arts, successful, productive, creative, and eventually sharing that with my children. I could almost see the oasis across the desert.

It was later that week when the doctors told me that Max was going to have to stay longer in the NICU than was anticipated. He ended up staying for five weeks. The doctors reassured us that his immature lungs needed time to develop, since he was born five weeks premature. They explained that the condition was common and that he would "grow out of it" as he reached his expected birth date. My husband and I joked with the doctors that Max was the largest baby in the NICU and he thoroughly enjoyed a team of women taking care of him.

As a mom with mild to moderate baseline anxiety, I felt that there was no better newborn care than a team of nurses and doctors providing around-the-clock monitoring. I remember that first visit to the NICU. I had slept a full night's sleep and showered, dried my hair, and stopped to get coffee on the way. I showed up to the unit, refreshed and ready to be with him. I sat there while he was in the incubator. He had tubes in his nose and he slept. I remember feeling guilty that he was agitated and uncomfortable from the tubes, and here I was feeling so comfortable after our birth experience. It should be me feeling the pain, anguish, and suffering, not my Max.

The nurses assured me that he would be okay, and that this was temporary. But I alleviated some of my concern for my newborn by working with the staff to make him more comfortable, and I brought him the coziest clothing items I could find. I stayed all day with him and held him as often as I could, bottle-fed and nursed, sang, and read books to him. Then, after a full day with him, I would pick up Jordan from daycare and take care of her at night and early mornings while my husband would go to spend time with Max.

I visited the NICU every day, giving Max whatever I could, enjoying him without being bogged down by the responsibilities of the newborn phase, and still being able to care for my toddler daughter. I left the hospital feeling like Supermom. Maybe it was the oxytocin from pumping and breastfeeding, or the fact that my husband and I were sleeping, regularly, every night. We had so much time to take care of our needs during those first five weeks that one evening I came home from visiting Max at the hospital and found my husband carefully tending to three mini planters of bonsai tree seedlings. If he couldn't take care of our son, he had to take care of something.

At the end of the fifth week, the doctors told us Max could come home. We were thrilled and also guiltily joked to each other that the vacation was over, remembering the early weeks of the newborn phase from Jordan. Of course, the day before we were supposed to bring him home from the hospital, Jordan developed a febrile illness. Nervous that Max would get sick too, I asked the doctors if he could stay in the NICU another couple of days until her illness resolved. Yes, you read that correctly. I asked the doctors if my son could extend his stay at the NICU, as if it were some posh baby resort that could simply extend the reservation. The attending looked at me like I had asked to give my baby a martini. I am pretty sure she never heard *any mother* ask for a longer stay in the NICU, and she simply replied, "We don't do that." The absurdity of that question is not lost on me now. However, at the time, it felt like a perfectly reasonable request.

I had prepared for the difficulty of the newborn phase as best as any mother could following his discharge from the hospital.

My foolproof plan included a night nurse to help with feedings for two weeks, continued care from our nanny for our high-energy toddler, and prescheduled family member visits. Mike planned to take two weeks off work to help with the transition from a one-baby to a two-baby household. For two months of my maternity leave, I organized coverage for my current patients so I could completely focus on my family. I organized a significant amount of instrumental support, including regularly dropped-off home-cooked meals made by my mother-in-law and a group of mommy best friends I could lean on for support. I set up my mental health care postdelivery, just in case. I would continue my weekly sessions with Dr. Nancy, and I lined up a psychiatrist for postpartum medication management, although I had never needed medication before. Nonetheless, I covered my bases. I had designed a postpartum plan to protect my brain, just as I would instruct my patients.

My postpartum plan was running smoothly until, four weeks after Max's discharge, a deadly global pandemic was looming.

For several weeks, my husband and I walked around our home like we forked an electric outlet, two hypervigilant deer in headlights. Mike was part of a nationwide physician's WhatsApp messaging group and got continuous updates about COVID-19. At the time, the virus was slaughtering Europe. With each alert of the app, an uneasiness stirred inside me parallel to the pandemic brewing overseas.

The only life raft I could cling to were the numbers that reflected children and babies were spared.

One morning, the ping of the notification shivered down my spine as I turned to my husband. "The virus is in Seattle," he said as he reminded me that we were two weeks behind Italy. There was discussion of doctors rationing care, which weighed heavily on my husband, as he "did not train for these types of ethical decisions. It's the stuff you read about in textbooks but never think it will actually happen." For weeks, Mike was attached to his phone, and I followed him around the house, waiting for follow-up texts.

My husband and I begged our parents and extended family to quarantine, sharing what seemed like insider information that our nation's news channels neglected. Our pleading was met with surprise. "Really? It's that bad?" some asked, while others were in denial, saying "It's not real; it's a hoax!"

And then the anxiety hit. I thought everyone was going to die. I had never been so terrified in my life. My brain was on fire. I did not sleep for five days straight. I lay awake planning how to protect my family from COVID. Max was just out of the NICU for lung-related issues. Every single safety net had holes the size of football fields. Every option was a double bind. I worried about one of us getting sick and spreading it to the entire household. If all of us were sick, who would take care of our babies and us? No one could help and risk exposure.

The beginning of COVID was a global trauma, and I knew we were not alone. Everyone was in the nightmare, together but separate. Parallel versions of *The Hunger Games*, every household for itself.

My worries spiraled. What if Mike got sick and *I* had to take care of an infant and a toddler all day and night with no sleep for weeks? What if I never slept again? Would I go insane? If I did go insane, how would I get emergency psychiatric care? I couldn't go to the hospital for psychiatric care because I couldn't risk exposure. How would I even get to the hospital if I was insane and couldn't drive? Ambulances were filled with COVID microbes. What if I was insane but was the only one physically well enough to take care of my babies? I know what can happen when you have an insane caretaker. I worried about being on the verge of experiencing postpartum psychosis. I knew all the statistics: although rare, postpartum psychosis occurs in one to two mothers for every 1,000 births. That postpartum psychosis can lead to infanticide (4 percent risk) and suicide (5 percent risk). What if I lost control of my mind? I still feel like I am here, but mothers are 23 times more likely to experience postpartum psychosis in the first month after birth. Although I was past that risk window, it was still early on and I was having sudden hormonal changes.

What if I unknowingly hurt my baby? What if I was so tired from not sleeping that I fell asleep and dropped him? I held on to the fact that 70 to 90 percent of new parents report intrusive and scary thoughts. That although I was having these thoughts, they were not necessarily indicative of any real danger.

Our house rule was "no one in, no one out." The night nurse left after two weeks. She couldn't come back if we needed her because she started her next job and was probably already exposed. We paid our nanny to take leave and keep herself safe. I couldn't hire the NICU nurses who offered to help because they were in and out of the hospital. We were alone. I was alone. I could not turn my brain off. I was stuck in a spiral that was propelled by a global pandemic and the hormonal shift of my recent decision to wean my son from breastfeeding more quickly than I would recommend and before knowing that we would be on lockdown long term.

Despite worrying we would all die from COVID-19, I did have the wherewithal to realize I was lucky that I married a man with different triggers. Mike's fears were centered on financial peril, such as his practice going under and nonessential surgeries being canceled. He imagined we would lose everything we worked so hard to build—financial stability, a home, a full life. He worried that he would be drafted to the front lines and contract COVID-19 from taking care of patients. He too was terrified.

We held each other at night, and I cried on his shoulder. He reassured me, saying that even if we got COVID, we would definitely not die. I reassured him and said that we would be fine financially no matter what. I lied. He lied. We tried to keep each other's heads above water. But underneath, I was drowning.

I could no longer pretend that I was okay. After another sleepless night, I headed down to the kitchen the next morning. The coffee pulled at me. I stared at it, carafe in hand. I was stuck in yet another spiral about getting COVID and not being able to take care of Jordan and Max when my eyes welled up with tears. My husband interrupted my daze. "I need you," he said. "Try to hold on to the present. We can get through this together." I looked up. I didn't even know he was in the kitchen. I wondered how long had he seen me. I quickly responded, "Don't worry. I'm not going anywhere. I am here with you!" While I meant it with everything in my soul, I was scared and uncertain that the rest of my brain and body would not follow suit.

I took the coffee upstairs, retreated to my closet, and closed the door. I remembered the acoustics in my closet being so good, it was the only place I could cry without Jordan hearing me. I texted my psychiatrist, Dr. Lane, "I am fully committed to taking medication." Having always been able to run myself out of any frustration or disappointment, I never thought that statement would come out of my mouth. She responded with an appointment time later that day.

In graduate school, I rotated on a consultation liaison service at a small community hospital. The service primarily provided psychiatric diagnostic assessments for any patient who presented in the emergency room. However, we would also get consults from other units of the hospital—neurology, intensive care, orthopedics. The position required me to assess and diagnose quickly and on my feet. As a result, I memorized over 40 mnemonic devices to recall symptoms of psychiatric disorders.

SIGECAPS was the mnemonic device for diagnosing major clinical depression. As I waited for Dr. Lane to call me, I stood in my closet, looking down at my feet, and slowly recited the acronym in my head. SIGECAPS: sleep, loss of interest, guilt, loss of energy, trouble concentrating, changes in appetite, psychomotor slowing, and suicidal ideation. Six out of eight positive symptoms were indicative of major depressive disorder.

My phone rang as I met criteria. "Hi, Nicole. How are you doing?"

Comforted by Dr. Lane's voice, I wanted to respond with a thoughtful, detailed explanation of symptoms. I wanted to tell her that I hadn't slept in five days and proclaim with clinical acumen that I thought you were supposed to start hallucinating after three. And that I had no other interests besides preventing my family from dying of COVID, so *yes* to loss of interest. I felt terribly guilty that I couldn't be present with my baby. That this morning I lay on the floor and cried about an unmade bed. That I thought of my own mother making a perfect bed, and what a great mother she is, and how I probably didn't tell her that enough, and I was a terrible daughter. Guilt.

I wanted to explain through my staccato thoughts that I had no energy and I wasn't sure how I was standing upright right now, given that I hadn't slept in five days, and did I mention I haven't slept in FIVE days?! In terms of concentration, the only thing I could concentrate on was COVID. Did that count? In that case, I had excellent concentration. For appetite, I could eat, but everything moved right through me because I PROBABLY HAVE COVID because gastrointestinal symptoms are SYMPTOMS OF COVID, and how can I know for sure that I don't have COVID and that I am not infecting my family as we speak?

My mind moved fast, but all I could actually say to Dr. Lane was, "Not. Good."

Then it occurred to me. I finally experienced psychomotor slowing—the seventh letter in that mnemonic device. My body could not catch up to my mind, and words left my mouth in slow motion. I have only seen psychomotor slowing one time in my clinical practice and a handful of times throughout my 10 years of graduate training. Your mind moves at regular speed, but your body has a slow paralysis, like a mini version of locked-in syndrome. It's what I imagine waking up midsurgery under anesthesia feels like, when you are too aware of what is going on but have no way to communicate it to your doctor.

Hunched over in my fatigue, I listened as Dr. Lane consoled me and went through her medication recommendations. The COVID pandemic was beginning to feel like a very real trauma developing, and I was watching it unfold. Flashes of Disney movies played in my mind—Jafar explaining to Aladdin, "Things are unraveling fast now, boyyyyyy!" and I could hear him warn me. An image from *Bambi* kept taunting me, a movie that just a month prior felt so comforting as I cuddled with Jordan and we awwwed together at baby Thumper. I became that panicked bird in the field, pacing around and shrieking about what is going to happen, so hysterical that she ends up prematurely darting in front of the hunter's shot.

I thought back to my days working on the burn unit at Johns Hopkins, when I was exposed to so many stories of patients' traumas. I was reminded of one of my colleagues, dear to me, who was investigating the relationship between heart rate and the development of PTSD following a severe burn injury. Turns out, there were gender differences where the higher the heart rate upon admission to the hospital and throughout their stay was related to greater PTSD symptoms at later points in time (e.g., one month, six months, 12 months) for women only.[29] It has been found that while men experience more trauma in general, women are more likely to experience PTSD after a traumatic incident. Women also have greater physiological reactivity after trauma compared to men. Discussions with my colleague following the findings in her research involved her next steps of potentially studying how a beta blocker could be administered to burn victims while being transported to the hospital. They were in the acute (early) stage of trauma, just like I was during those early weeks of the pandemic. The hypotheses for the research was that the beta blocker could blunt the physiological trauma response early on and thus could potentially protect patients from developing full-blown PTSD. I had thought about this frequently during the previous few weeks. Actually, the thought kept repeating itself in my brain, that I *had* to protect my brain. I was too aware, taking in too much of the experience of trauma in real time. Ultimately, this was the final convincing rationale for me to take medication for emotional reactivity during this period. It was no coincidence that my mind was searching for sources of comfort in trauma and my colleague, my friend, and a nurturing maternal figure in my life appeared.

I knew what I needed to do. I needed to blunt my own trauma response so that I would prevent PTSD later. I had never taken medication before. However, during these postpartum days, the decision came more promptly than I expected.

Dr. Lane prescribed me a sleep aid and low-dosage SSRI. I continued to meet frequently with my psychotherapist as well. Dr. Nancy advised to me to make sure I got outside every day for a walk to reset my circadian rhythm and continued to do light therapy, and she worked with me to shift my distorted thoughts and obsessions during this time. I did everything she told me. She checked in with me daily, and for all of this I am eternally grateful.

On day nine, I was sleeping for hours at a time and feeling relief. It was the scariest nine days of my life, wondering where I would end up—a psychiatric nightmare or a return to normalcy? I celebrated the first morning I awoke no longer gripped with fear of how I would get through the day.

Hindsight is 20/20. For me, being able to recognize and diagnose early symptoms of postpartum depression and an OCD crisis while getting real treatment from the mental health team I established prior to delivery helped me recover quickly. It is much easier to treat depression when caught early. Mothers are Oscar-worthy in their attempts to mask and compensate for their suffering while taking care of a newborn. However, everyone benefits from getting treatment. Everyone. Sometimes, as mothers, we are not aware of how much we impact the entire household. It is often not until a crisis hits that it becomes apparent that the primary caregiver is the center of the village.

It's not just mothers; it's fathers too. Current research indicates 8 to 10 percent of fathers experience postpartum depression. There are many explanations of why there is a discrepancy between postpartum depression and anxiety in men and women, from lack of hormone changes to not being the primary caregiver. Another potential explanation of why men don't experience PPDA as frequently as women could also be because men may be more incisive about taking care of their own needs, which may in turn prevent PPDA.

There are many reasons why my postpartum mental health vulnerability evolved into a mental health crisis. First, the postpartum period is widely known as a very vulnerable time for maternal mental health. That means mothers and primary caregivers are more likely to develop mental health conditions, such as postpartum depression, anxiety, OCD, psychosis, and other conditions, compared to the general population. At baseline, due to my personal history of anxiety, I was also vulnerable to develop worse anxiety during the postpartum period.

In addition, the risk increases after each pregnancy and delivery. So, while therapy worked to manage my anxiety after my first pregnancy, the second bout was much more severe. This is not always the case, and again hindsight is 20/20. However, knowing the likelihood of me experiencing another postpartum episode, more severe than the last, prompted me to have my mental health team intact and ready to treat. I advise the same for all my patients.

I am reminded of one of my patients, Mia, who had a complicated history of bipolar I disorder. She contacted me one month before she was due with her first baby. Mia had a preference for managing her bipolar disorder without medication and had successfully done so for years. Over a decade of managing her condition was interrupted by only one manic episode that required medication intervention. I agreed to take her on as a patient in my practice under one condition: I required her to have an evaluation with a psychiatrist to establish care before she delivered and to schedule her follow-up visit at three weeks postpartum.

We collaboratively devised a postpartum mental health plan, and I wanted to support her preference for not taking medication. However, I held on to the understanding that while she may not have preferred medication, I was the expert in the room. As my patient, if she needed treatment, she would get treatment. I had her sign a release form so that her psychiatrist and I could communicate about her mental health needs.

How to Manage a Maternal Mental Health Crisis

- The postpartum period is a period of vulnerability to mental health symptoms.
- There is an increased risk for mothers to develop perinatal depression, anxiety, psychosis, and OCD postpartum.
- With each additional pregnancy and delivery, the risk of postpartum depression and anxiety increases if you had a prior episode.
- Meet with your mental health provider before giving birth to discuss risk based on your personal health history.

I also communicated with her partner. Mia agreed to bring her into session as I provided psychoeducation about the signs and symptoms of bipolar disorder. I also discussed a plan with them about how to preserve my patient's sleep. Sleep and exercise had been two of the main mood management strategies that have helped Mia's mood remain stable for years. She was well aware of the cost of playing with less sleep, as it triggered the manic episode she had six years prior.

This is not uncommon. There is a reason the latest *Textbook of Women's Reproductive Mental Health* strongly advises to protect mothers' sleep. Sleep disturbance is a risk factor for many mental health conditions, including postpartum depression and anxiety. Unfortunately, taking care of a newborn is synonymous with disturbed sleep. Many mothers (and fathers) find this to be incredibly stressful. For primary caregivers, it can make symptoms worse and lead to clinical levels of depression and anxiety. Knowing this, I spent two entire sessions with Mia discussing the importance of sleep, normalizing and preparing for disrupted sleep, and strategies for improving and preserving sleep. Given her previously established diagnosis of bipolar disorder and disrupted sleep precipitating mania, it was of the utmost importance to preserve her mental health.

After much discussion, Mia's partner agreed to a postpartum plan, which included that her partner would take over the middle-of-the-night feedings. This was so Mia could get at least one stretch of five to six hours of sleep. I discussed other ways of improving sleep during the newborn phase, which include "resting" while the baby rests and reducing stimulation. I did not pressure her to "sleep when the baby sleeps." While that is a nice idea, it often just adds unrealistic expectations and mothers get even more frustrated when they have difficulty falling asleep during brief nap windows.

Instead, I advise them to get an eye mask and lie in a dark, cool room. I instruct them to listen to relaxation recordings and practice deep breathing. If they fall asleep, great (oftentimes, this helps them fall asleep even for a catnap), and if they don't, they are at least less stimulated and more rested. They are not worried or frustrated by the fact that they didn't sleep. Instead, I reframe their brief nap or rest as a restorative activity. Then we continue to problem-solve about how to work toward the goal of getting more actual sleep.

Mia and her partner stuck to the postpartum plan in the early weeks and things remained stable. However, my patient's milk supply was low and she struggled with breastfeeding. She ended up supplementing with formula, but that quickly became overwhelming for her. She made the decision to stop breastfeeding and switch to formula, and the weaning was much less gradual than I would recommend for mood stability.

We see an increase in PPDA after stopping breastfeeding and also after delivery if mothers choose not to or cannot breastfeed. Because I am aware of this trajectory, I carefully monitored her symptoms. The first week, there were no symptoms of mania. The second week, she started feeling more energized and was beginning to brainstorm new creative projects that were coming to mind. She was aware of this "energy" and, behaviorally, we had to slow things down for her. She had to work diligently on reducing stimulation. The third week, she admitted that she started feeling paranoid when she was home alone with her baby and thought that the mailman and package delivery workers were going to try to enter her home.

All along this course, I remained in contact with Mia's psychiatrist, and we shared our diagnostic impressions and symptom reports weekly. It became clear that the train was already headed down the track and that she would need medication intervention to slow it down. The session that week had been focused on processing her feelings about needing medication at this moment to protect her brain. We did not want to wait and see what full-blown mania would entail. The increase of severity of symptoms and frequency, along with her history, allowed her to get treatment very early on and prevent a full-blown manic episode. The psychiatrist and I also worked collaboratively with the patient to get her off the medication when she was stable for a long enough period of time, knowing that was her preference.

Another evidence-based treatment I like to provide early on in postpartum is behavioral activation for depression. In simple terms, behavioral activation consists of scheduling pleasurable activities and teaching patients how to increase pleasure, in order to reduce avoidance, mood-driven behaviors, and increase goal-directed behaviors to improve mood. In strict behavioral activation, I would be helping my patients monitor their activities, rate pleasure and positive results from behavior, track mood, and then create firm schedules filled with various activities that are correlated with boosting their mood. There would be charts and graphs and analyses. However, new moms don't have time for charts and graphs. In early postpartum, it is also very difficult for mothers to have a set schedule. Between the baby's unpredictable feedings and sleep, nothing is routine. During this time, I adapt the behavioral activation strategies for my patients.

First, I explain to my patients that they will have to be curious about what will bring them pleasure after having a baby. They will also have to think small, given time and location barriers. The behavioral activation treatment manual includes 320 activities, most of which would not apply to new mothers. Plus, when we become mothers, besides identity changes, the things we used to enjoy may also change. So it is worth taking time to come up with a comprehensive list of practical activities that bring you pleasure and apply to this unique time period.

Your brain, the pathways, the neurotransmitters, the physical parts—it all changes. Your hormones, your psyche, your relationships—all change. Your interests, your schedule, your needs, your pleasures—ALL CHANGE. The reward center of your brain is the striatum, and it is dictated by several dopamine pathways. The striatum is responsible for producing feelings of reward and pleasure. When I became a mother, I was surprised to find that there were actual physiological changes associated with changes in pleasure. Research indicates that there are specific anatomical changes in the pleasure center of the brain that are responsible. In sum, volume in the striatum decreases during pregnancy and after birth, which is positively associated with increases in striatum activation to baby cues. In other words, the greater the reduction in the reward center of the brain, the greater the activation of pleasure response to your baby.

My reward pathways are now deeply reinforced by the simple joys that accompany my love for my children. Perhaps I need less because I have so much more. When I try to access some of those old pleasures, they just don't hit the mark. Not that I can't enjoy a nice vacation, a night out, or skiing down a mountain on a bluebird day. It's just that the pleasure center in my brain has expanded and the dopamine hits from interactions with my baby are off the charts.

So I work with my patients to come up with a list of practical, pleasurable activities that they like to do, and I encourage them to keep it with them as a daily checklist. Perhaps it is only three things, perhaps it is a dozen. Maybe it is meditating, listening to a brief podcast, smelling their baby's hair, rocking their baby for pleasure, a brief walk, doing some yoga poses, reading, or an episode of a travel show or guilty pleasure sitcom. Here's another tip: keep a portable folding chair in your car. Next time you take a break, head to a peaceful spot—a lake, a pond, the ocean, a peaceful wooded area—and sit in peace. Listen to nature. I also encourage them to remind themselves that they need to seize the opportunity to protect their mental health when a moment frees up. These activities can help you reset. Also, I encourage them to not be hard on themselves if they miss a day, or if they only get to one activity. Depression is not like the flu, where you lay in bed and wait until you feel better. Waiting it out makes it worse. You have to make yourself do things that bring you pleasure to get the benefits of the mood-boosting activities.

Another evidence-based recommendation I make to my patients is to do light therapy. Northern Light Technologies has a desk lamp that delivers bright light therapy. Bright light therapy is low-cost, convenient, and has been shown to be effective for reducing symptoms of seasonal and nonseasonal depression. There has been limited research on light therapy for perinatal mood disorders, but some studies show it can be effective for reducing symptoms of postpartum depression.[30] It is important that you try light therapy under the supervision of a postpartum mental health specialist because there is some research that indicates it can exacerbate symptoms of bipolar disorder. With light therapy, it is recommended that you sit 18 to 24 inches away from the lamp in front of you on a desk or table for 20 to 30 minutes per day. That's all you need. You can do light therapy while you pump, listen to a podcast or music, or fold baby clothes.

When I think of my patients with postpartum depression, anxiety, OCD, and other perinatal mental health symptoms, I consider Mia's story, and others', treatment successes. Success is not the absence of mental health conditions and symptoms. We have little control over whether our brains will suffer from postpartum depression and anxiety or not. It was extremely helpful for me to frame my own mental health postpartum, as well as my patients', as "my brain likes to do this thing postpartum . . ." It allows us to get distance from the diagnosis and prevents us from getting caught up in a label or stigma. While perinatal mental health awareness is improving, unfortunately, some level of stigma still exists.

Postpartum depression and anxiety actually impact your perspective. We tend to have more critical views of ourselves when we are depressed and anxious. We view ourselves as failing, terrible mothers, doing something wrong, or not fit for this role because we are more depressed and anxious. The problem is not the content of the thoughts; the problem is the depression and anxiety. That needs treatment. With treatment, you can more clearly see the disorder for what it is, separate from who you are as a mother going through a really challenging phase. As mothers, we often get lost in our depressive and anxious thoughts, thinking they are accurate when really they are symptoms of underlying medical conditions that need treatment. Get treatment.

SNAPSHOT

How to Manage a Maternal Mental Health Crisis

- It is your job to protect your brain.
- Have a partner or support person take over a night feeding to give the biological mother or primary caregiver a longer stretch of sleep she can count on (five to six hours, with the majority of hours before midnight for more restorative sleep).
- Adopt this saying if you have a history of postpartum: "My brain likes to do this thing postpartum. Here is what I can do if my brain does it again." List steps and plan with your mental health team. Share the plan with your partner.
- Postpartum mental health conditions distort your perception. We tend to think we are failing as mothers or doing something wrong. The problem is not the content of these statements. Think of these statements as symptoms of potential underlying perinatal depression or anxiety, and discuss them with your mental health care provider.
- Current research indicates 8 to 10 percent of fathers experience postpartum depression as well. Fathers and other caregivers should seek mental health treatment if indicated.

PART III

How to Go from Surviving to
Thriving in Early Motherhood

11

HOW TO SELF-DIRECT MATERNAL NEUROPLASTICITY

"When they go low, we go high."
—MICHELLE OBAMA, FORMER FIRST LADY AND MOTHER OF TWO

Now that we have gotten through how to remove some of the major roadblocks in motherhood, let's review and get to more specific strategies that can promote greater enhancement and optimal functioning. Psychology is not just about treating mental illness, it is also about promoting resilience. When symptoms are managed or when there are no deficits, we can still improve our functioning, enhance quality of life, and thrive.

I knew my brain would recover from postpartum, but I could not have imagined coming out the other side thriving, especially during a global pandemic. We know that pregnancy and maternal brain development is riddled with land mines, from increased inflammatory markers necessary to protect from infection and increased sensitivity to threats, to decreases in grey matter, which can increase maternal vulnerability to postpartum depression and anxiety.[31]

I was well versed in the risks, but no one spoke to me about the incredible potential of my new mommy brain. In fact, public knowledge of mommy brain is limited to an archaic at best, and destructive at worst, representation alluding to "forgetfulness" and "clumsy thought." Each unprecedented challenge in the pandemic forced me to figure it out—because I was a mother. I did not realize that rising to such incredible challenges would ultimately fine-tune my brain and make me better than ever.

You now know from reading this book that the mommy brain undergoes immense neural plasticity with potentially enormous benefits. To summarize, a proliferation of cells and networks emerge and reorganize themselves to orient to child-rearing. Anything not of the utmost importance to child-rearing gets discarded in our brains; cells acting as little Marie Kondos of the mind. Thus, that mommy brain moment of trying to remember someone's name in favor of a vigilant eye on junior on the playground is only nature's way of keeping the species alive. There is no greater period of physiological, hormonal, or psychological changes in such a short period of time than with pregnancy. In comparison, the physiological changes occur more quickly, with the greatest changes beginning in pregnancy and in the early months postpartum. The psychological and identity transformation is slower and takes much longer to adjust to motherhood. These processes are occurring at the same time, but mothers often think that they should sync up. What I want mothers to understand is that just because the physical changes may occur faster, the psychological changes likely need time to catch up.

During pregnancy, the brain reorganizes itself to support the development of the fetus and to care for an infant after birth. Neural plasticity refers to the proliferation of synapses and new connections that are developed to best support tending to an infant. In other words, necessary parts improve their functioning and unnecessary parts shrink or decrease in functioning. Think of your brain as an elaborate highway system. Those old highways are no longer needed, so they tend to decay or become overgrown with trees and weeds. Your brain develops new pathways of motherhood, similar to breaking through jungle vines with a machete to create a path and then ultimately to create a clear and efficient highway. In the transition to motherhood, it seems like there is a great opportunity to work with the system to tweak the physiological processes (i.e., neural plasticity) already in motion to your advantage. Neural plasticity can be harnessed and influenced by therapy, challenges, life events, trauma, and other external factors.

In motherhood, the evolution of neuroplastic changes based on the mother's experiences with the baby is known as experience-dependent plasticity. Katherine Ellison's 2006 book, *The Mommy Brain: How Motherhood Makes Us Smarter*, speaks to the many ways becoming a mother makes our brain more efficient; helps us adapt to challenges; and engages us in intense, baby-led training for optimal functioning. Ellison told me recently that "in any given moment, a mother is asked to nurture, protect, negotiate, decipher, solve, repair, mitigate, bond with her baby, and manage her own emotion regulation." The mother is the object that serves to meet all the infant's demands, as the infant is completely dependent on the mother. However, the mother is not an endless resource, though she is tasked with responding to the urgency of the infant's demands (e.g., the infant is not aware of the mother being separate and having separate needs).

I use the term *relentless* with my patients, as a baby is constantly demanding for their needs to be met. Mark Epstein, MD, author of *The Zen of Therapy*, states, "A baby wants food and closeness and soothing and excitement and contact and stimulation, and he or she wants it without regard for a mother's feelings, and he or she wants it now." As the mother rises to the challenge, the mother is developing and fine-tuning her skill set as she meets these demands. That is not to say that it is perfect—it isn't and should not be. In fact, psychologist Donald Winnicott coined the term "good enough mother" for a reason. A mother does not have to be perfect to be good. Epstein discusses that the mother will actually teach the dependent infant and child, in developmentally appropriate and gradual ways, that the mother cannot meet all the baby's needs all the time and all at once. The infant will experience momentary disappointment, and it is through this disappointment that repair can occur. Epstein further emphasizes that the "cycle of rupture and repair" is necessary and evident in all interpersonal relationships. While the role of being a mother is ruthless, the ability for the maternal brain to meet the demands of the child allows the maternal brain to become sharper, smarter, and more psychologically advanced.

In prior generations, the majority of maternal care included washing cloth diapers, making food from scratch, cleaning, gardening, and more stay-at-home mothers engaging in minute-by-minute physical care. Today, motherhood is much more cerebral; we have more physical resources, and more mothers are engaged in the workforce. Modern stay-at-home mothers and working mothers are more involved in planning, negotiating, and organizing care, play dates, mommy-and-me activities, and other brain-powered tasks, versus tilling the land with their offspring. Regardless, mothers' personal activities are critical to their mental health.

Kelly Lambert, PhD, professor of behavioral neuroscience at the University of Richmond, has been studying maternal neuroplasticity in rodents for decades. Lambert's latest research investigates how enriched environments affect mental health, impacting the brain by promoting neuroplasticity (how neurons are formed in the brain) and hippocampal and spatial memory functioning. The pandemic has forced mothers and fathers alike to be creative and figure out ways to enrich their home environments. Lambert coined the term *behaviorceuticals* and speaks to the limitations of medication on brain plasticity. In other words, medications can help promote brain plasticity; however, she believes it's the behavioral changes that can do more, go further, and promote longer-lasting plasticity with and without the aid of medication. In parenthood, the brain plasticity is further propelled by rising to the challenges of parenthood; regulating your own emotions to effectively and creatively problem-solve; and cultivating positive emotions, such as joy. I'll speak more about the positive emotions and their benefits to the mind later in this chapter.

In Lambert's books, *Lifting Depression: A Neuroscientist's Hands-On Approach to Activating Your Brain's Healing Power* and *Well-Grounded: The Neurobiology of Rational Decisions*, she speaks to the evolution of the maternal brain and how our ancestors used to do more hands-on work. Doctors used to prescribe knitting to their patients to treat depression, an effort-based reward system pertaining to the connection between the personal and physical labor. In one of her studies on rats, the rats that were able to dig up their cereal treats were more protected against developing depression-like symptoms. Lambert translates that finding to modern-day mothers— when so many things are out of our control in early motherhood, it's crucial to introduce, maintain, or develop an activity that can help you regain a sense of control. Even more so, the activity should be something that is physical and uses your hands. Eighty percent of neurons are located in the brain's cerebellum, which is responsible for motor coordination. Using your hands in an activity engages the cortex and bilateral brain spheres. So much of the real estate in your brain is dedicated to moving. When you don't use it, you lose it. When so much real estate is going unused, the brain becomes vulnerable to depression.

If we can use what we know about how to increase, direct, and improve plasticity, we can apply the same tenets to the maternal brain. Early on, I encourage mothers to take up a postpartum activity that uses their hands, based on Lambert's research. It may seem like a challenging time to take up a new hobby, but try to think of it in small steps. For example, you can easily order a child's craft kit to try, like a loom to make potholders, a beginner crochet kit, gimp or string to make bracelets, or yarn and straws to do straw weaving (YouTube it—so easy!). These crafts have safe materials, are simple enough for kids to do them, and also keep your hands busy and thus exercise the motor area of your brain, which can be protective for anxiety and depression. Indeed, research has shown that crocheting and knitting can increase serotonin and reduce stress. Plus, the repetitive movements used in these activities can be self-soothing.

Rick Hanson, PhD, a clinical psychologist and author of *Hardwiring Happiness*, explains self-directed neuroplasticity and ways to improve neural networks related to calm, happiness, and peace. Isn't that what a mother needs the most, improved ways to feel calmer, happier, and more peaceful? In psychology, we understand that it is much easier for negative experiences to form neural networks in our brain. This is because our brain is wired to protect us from danger. When we have negative experiences, the memories are seared and etched in our brains for protection. It is much more difficult to cultivate neural networks in our brain from positive experiences. However, we can do this if we practice. Like a skill set, the more we practice, the better we get.

Self-directed neuroplasticity refers to cultivating neural networks, and there are several strategies in Hanson's book and in the field of positive psychology to help foster this ability. In other words, by using the strategies I will discuss shortly, you have the power to actually change your brain at a neural level. When becoming a mother, your brain is already set in motion to do this, but the focus is for the benefit of child-rearing. This is necessary. What I am suggesting is that you ride this wave of neuroplasticity and use it to your advantage to help yourself during this process. Your brain will more easily focus on the baby, and it's easy to shift brain power in that direction. We can become more resilient, less stressed, and happier caregivers if we also build some neural networks that benefit ourselves at this critical time.

In regard to self-directed neuroplasticity and the potential to thwart maladaptive conditions, it's important to consider its role in helping to prevent the development of postpartum depression. A recent study found that women suffering from postpartum depression had lower plasma levels of brain-derived neurotrophic factor (BDNF) compared to their nondepressed counterparts.[32] BDNF levels also rose in the depression-recovery group. BDNF plays a major role in plasticity by increasing synaptic activity, binding receptors in neural networks, and fostering neuron proliferation. It is well established that physical exercise increases BDNF concentrations and promotes plasticity.[33] If we can increase plasticity by using self-directed techniques, there may be potential to reduce the risk of developing postpartum depression. This is a good question for research trials that unfortunately has not been addressed yet. I did, however, find one study that examined the results of pregnant women over the age of 35 who participated in an exercise program, and results yielded higher levels of BDNF and other markers of plasticity in their offspring.[34] However, they did not examine BDNF levels in the mothers, which I would encourage for future research.

It is imperative to get treatment for mental health conditions postpartum. Left untreated, the conditions can work against the efforts suggested here to improve neuroplastic processes. Real mental health treatment works to change maladaptive networks in the brain and build stronger networks by providing corrective emotional experiences through the relationship with the therapist and other interpersonal relationships, changing distorted thought patterns, and increasing healthy behaviors. In therapy sessions, I tell my patients we are rewiring the brain.

Here are some more ways we can work with the neuroplastic changes that are occurring in the maternal brain instead of fighting them. First, establish care with a mental health care provider for therapy and a psychiatrist for medication management *before* you give birth. You do not have to determine whether your worry, distress, or other symptoms are a "normal" part of motherhood. The professionals can do that, so let them do their jobs. Perinatal mental health conditions can get in the way of adaptive brain changes that occur in early motherhood. We not only want to nurture the adaptive changes that are naturally occurring, but we also want to remove any obstacles that would get in their way.

SNAPSHOT

How to Self-Direct Maternal Neuroplasticity

- Medications can promote brain plasticity, but behavioral changes can do more, go further, and promote longer-lasting plasticity.
- In motherhood, try to maintain, introduce, or develop an activity that allows you to regain control.
- Motherhood is more cerebral than ever. Doing something active with your hands or motor neurons can help protect your brain against developing depression.
- Get treatment for mental health symptoms, including depression and anxiety, to help your brain optimally benefit from the transition to motherhood.
- Therapy can rewire the brain.

Therapy is like building new roads in your brain and letting old highways dissipate. I steer my patients to avoid the old roads that reinforce maladaptive thought patterns and work with them to create new roads. This is especially important during motherhood, when so many new neural networks are being formed. *It's all new learning.* One of the most important ways I help my patients create new roads is with the bridge "and" between two contradictory states, also known as cognitive dissonance. I love my baby AND I need to take a break. I want my baby to have the best nutrition AND breastfeeding is sacrificing my mental health. I want to tend to my baby's every need AND I would like to go back to work. I have needs AND my baby has needs. Tending to my needs will ultimately serve my baby because I will feel less stressed, be more present, and be able to problem-solve more effectively.

In the field of neuroplasticity, it is often said that "neurons that fire together, wire together." Holding these dialectical statements together is an example of extending this line of thinking. In the maternal brain there is room to add the "and" statement pertaining to your own needs in conjunction with concern for your baby. By more readily accepting many opposing diametric truths and practicing holding these truths simultaneously early on, you will force new neural networks to form that contain both your needs and your baby's needs.

Another premise that Hanson discusses in his book, *Hardwiring Happiness*, is to lean in to pleasure. I find this strategy particularly helpful to offset the many not-so-enjoyable moments of motherhood. As I mentioned in the beginning pages of this book, parents who are well beyond the early phases of child-rearing can look back with a sense of nostalgia and encourage new parents to "enjoy every moment." This is impossible. However, what you can do to offset those moments when your toddler just will not get dressed, or your baby wakes for the third time in the night, or a heated sibling fight breaks out, is to make those beautiful moments that come in between much bigger.

Every parent knows what I am talking about: those early-morning cuddles, those "I love you, Mommys," and those big smoochy kisses. Those moments when your baby smiles at you or begins to take their first steps, or your toddler says something remarkably intuitive, or when you all have giggle attacks together on the floor. It's those moments you have to magnify, hold on to, and enlarge. Imagine you will be that parent in 20 years, looking back with nostalgia, and wanting to tell the future generations to enjoy these moments. Build up your bank of big moments to draw from. You'll have more to hold on to as the grip on your children loosens. Plus, in the present, it will help buffer the challenging moments.

As I mentioned, as a new mom, your pleasure system will change.

Research supports that breastfeeding can be more gratifying than cocaine on the maternal rodent brain. Your new mom brain is also wired to wait for the other shoe to drop. Drop that habit. Self-directed neuroplasticity would say to increase that pleasure as much as you can.[35] For example, as you are rocking your baby, smell your baby's skin, feel the softness of your baby's head on your chest, play soothing music, envision your baby growing into a healthy adult and completing life's milestones. Then think about yourself as a mother and what type of mother you hope to be. Perhaps this involves healing your own mother wound. Think about what you are grateful for in this moment with your baby. As you think these thoughts about yourself and simultaneously engage your senses with your baby, new neurons will fire together and wire together, strengthening that pleasure and ultimately buffering against the stresses of motherhood. Let negative thoughts come and go, without judgment, as if they are just passing through. You can ask yourself when an intrusive, negative, or anxious thought comes to mind, "Do I want to strengthen this neural network or erase it from my memory?" Most likely, you will want those negative thoughts to weaken, and you have to work to redirect your mind back to pleasure. Engaging your senses can help bring you back to the present moment and gratification at hand. Spoil yourself in the pleasure of the moment. Your neurons will thank you.

In psychology, the advantage of cultivating positive emotions is supported by the Broaden-and-Build theory. Barbara Fredrickson, social psychologist and author of the book *Positivity*, developed the Broaden-and-Build theory. This theory suggests that positive emotions serve to broaden mindsets, while negative emotions tend to narrow these same cognitive processes. Positive emotions have an immediate effect on expanding one's outlook, and over time they can take on a more permanent, health-promoting role by fostering a greater breadth of resources, improving problem-solving and coping, and developing a greater ability to draw from those resources in times of need.

When I think about the emotional experiences of motherhood, I am reminded of a recent interaction. I visited one of my best friends the other day, and we spent time catching up. She is the type of friend who, no matter how much time has gone by or how long it has been since we have seen each other, we pick up where we left off without skipping a beat.

I walked into her house, and it was so quiet you could hear a pin drop. I was confused since she is a mother of two young boys, and I am quite used to them running around and chasing each other or throwing footballs at each other when I visit.

"This is what happens when your children get older," she reassured me. "They don't need you. They are off in their rooms, playing video games with their friends." It happened to be her older son's birthday that day, and I realized it had been at least a year since I had visited.

"But the level of worry stays the same," she continued. I knew exactly what she was talking about.

I told her a story. The other day, Mike was going to take Max to daycare and Jordan to school, which he usually does every Thursday. They were being particularly difficult that morning, and I was trying to move them along so that Mike wouldn't be late for work. I finally got them in the car, and as they drove off I mouthed to Mike, "See ya later" (adding "suckers" in my head), followed by a happy dance in the driveway. I headed back into the kitchen to bask in my gloriously empty house and drink my coffee. Then I had an automatic thought and immediately ruined my moment of freedom with guilt. What if they all get killed in a car crash on the way to school? Was it worth it, Nicole? There I was, daring to enjoy a cup of coffee, and my family is going to die.

My best friend told me a similar story. "Last week I had to run a last-minute errand, and I asked Matt to pick up Brady from his football practice. I imagined Brady with neither of us there watching his practice and then getting tackled and suffering a traumatic brain injury. I literally said to myself, this one decision could change our whole lives forever." She paused and then asked me, "Do you think we are the only ones who think like this?"

I informed her that no, I think lots of mothers think like this. In fact, I had just finished rereading Brené Brown's book, *The Gifts of Imperfection*. She speaks about this topic all the time. Her famous quote is, "The most terrifying emotion is joy." Brown expanded and explained that she had given a parenting talk to a group of moms and told the audience that terror often follows moments of joy. She then asked the audience, "How often do you stand over your children and think about how much you love them and then immediately imagine something terrible happening to them?" After a moment of silence from the audience, she said she could start to hear sobs from some women in the back of the room and someone shouting, "Yes! Why do we do this?!"

Brown further explained that we feel most vulnerable in our moments of joy, and that terror helps us "prepare" for the fact that the thing we love most can be taken away from us. However, she explains, the preparation for terror is futile. Nothing can prepare you for tragedy or dampen that experience. She then offered the antidote to those moments of terror: gratitude. Specifically, she recommends leaning in to the moments of joy harder by practicing gratitude.

It got me thinking about mother brains and how to offer more strategies for leaning in to joy. When we become mothers, our brain system goes through so many changes to orient to the baby. I believe this is also what is happening in these moments of terror: we are wired to "protect" our children. But joy is not protective in any way. Joy does not help us scan the environment for danger. In fact, joy does the opposite. Joy is acceptance and being present in the moment and experiencing the complete happiness of being suspended in time. There is no future to worry about in joy. This does nothing to help the baby. However, it is vital for the mother. These moments are what make it all worth it—the way the universe shows us how big our hearts can expand, how much we can possibly love a child, infinitely more than we imagined. So, to expand on Brown's suggestions to practice gratitude, I also suggest leaning in to joy more. There is no downside to this. Practice mindfulness and increase the pleasure in the moment. Ask yourself, "How can I possibly create more joy in this moment?"

First, take some deep belly breaths and ground yourself in the present moment. What are you seeing? Hearing? Feeling? Smelling? Tasting? Is there anything bringing you pleasure in this moment? Maybe you smell your baby's shampoo on their head, or play a fun song, or do a silly dance with them, or point out the clouds. Try to expand these moments of joy. Imagine you are trying to heighten your senses and amplify the experience. What can you add to make it last longer, make it more enjoyable, or enhance the sensations further? Can you add a warm blanket to snuggle up to your baby while smelling her hair? Can you play soothing spa music and give your baby a gentle massage with baby lotion? Can you do something for yourself, like listen to a book, watch a movie or show while feeding the baby and maybe snacking on dark chocolate? When you rock your baby, make up a story about their future that you would like to envision and play out the details in your mind. Allow yourself to feel vulnerable and scared that the moment feels too good and try to ignore the "when is the other shoe going to drop?" reaction to joy.

Our babies are better at cultivating joy because they do not yet have the prefrontal cortex to filter their behavior. They are natural joy seekers. For example, when I sing "The Wheels on the Bus" or read a *Llama Llama* book to my son, Max, he immediately nuzzles up against me, sticks his two fingers in his mouth, and begins sucking. This boy knows how to increase pleasure. He decides that he is going to make this experience of mommy singing or reading to him even more pleasurable by adding his soothing behavior to the mix. Several times, he has gathered not one, not two, but three pillows to rest on as he is experiencing story time. Max is a smart boy. Be like Max.

Another strategy I like to encourage is to allow yourself to approach motherhood with curiosity, flexibility, and empathy. As you make mistakes, be compassionate with yourself. Be curious about how that could go differently the next time. As you complete each new task, integrate it within yourself. For example, "Wow, I figured out how to soothe my baby by rocking up and down with him and rubbing his back gently. That's great problem-solving for someone who's never done this thing before." That way, you are giving yourself credit and incorporating value for yourself into what you are doing. Remember, it does not have to be perfect to be okay. By tending to your own needs, you are putting a placeholder in for your baby to tend to their own needs as they grow older, which is the optimal way to facilitate your baby's development.

Taken together, this research highlights the power of the maternal brain to become more optimally fine-tuned for child-rearing. This is an incredible opportunity to take advantage of the neurological gifts of plasticity and infuse mother-focused needs. If you can learn how to respond and become more attuned to baby cues, you can also think about becoming more attuned to your own internal cues. If you can discard what is not necessary for child-rearing, this is also an optimal time to discard what is no longer serving *you*. The maternal brain is primed and in the best shape for learning. This is an optimal time to integrate other material that can be learned, such as learning how to better care for yourself; learning about your own psychological constitution; learning about who you are in this new role and what type of parent you want to be; learning about your own triggers and how you were mothered and parented; learning in therapy; learning about your own needs; learning how to make space for yourself; and learning how to cultivate creativity, fun, and flexibility in this demanding phase. If we plant these seeds

before a mother gives birth, before the chaos ensues, we can better prepare mothers to understand that the baby is important and the mother
equally so. What will make you a better mother is digging into meeting
your own needs so you can better take care of your baby. The strategies
I recommend will help prepare you to think about your own needs, and
how that will help you be a better mother. You have plasticity on your
side to help with the baby stuff, and you can ride that plasticity and steer
it to include your own needs as well.

As I mentioned earlier, exercise promotes neurogenesis (how neurons are formed in the brain). Expanding upon the importance of
movement, exercise is nature's antidepressant. But mothers often have
trouble finding time to exercise. What I would think about is shifting
your perspective on exercise. It may not look like that HIIT class you
used to attend. Perhaps now it's a 20-minute walk around the block,
pushing the stroller. Or a series of stretches while wearing the baby
carrier. Whatever it is, protect a slot of time dedicated to some form
of exercise.

Physical travel also promotes neuroplasticity. When I spoke with
Lambert about her latest research project and investigating this notion
of "travel" in rodent brains, Lambert stated that she and her lab want to
better understand how enriched environments impact mental health.
She stated that they created a sort of Disneyland for their lab rats to be
able to travel back and forth between their living quarters. Travel also
promotes neurogenesis and hippocampal and spatial memory functioning. It got me thinking, *How can we adapt this notion of "travel" for
moms of infants and toddlers when the ability to physically travel is limited?*
Some ideas we discussed were planning a vacation, subscribing to travel
magazines and anticipating future trips, watching documentaries on
new places, and, if there are resources, splurging for or using a treadmill
that lets you run through a video-guided tour of the Alps. Lambert
called this a "double dose," as it would be exercising and "traveling."

How to Self-Direct Maternal Neuroplasticity

- Exercise is nature's antidepressant. Even if it is just a 20-minute walk. Your exercise preferences may change when you become a mom. Schedule exercise in your calendar.
- You can "travel." Watch travel documentaries, plan a vacation and itinerary, explore hotel options, subscribe to a travel magazine, read travel blogs, or purchase home treadmill equipment and use the nature feature when you exercise.
- Engage in effort-based reward behaviors and use your hands. For example, color in a coloring book, paint, garden, cook a meal, or knit. Schedule the 20-minute activity in your calendar. This will allow you to have a space where you can feel in control.
- Bridge "and" between two contradictory states in motherhood. Neurons that fire together, wire together.
- I love my baby AND I dislike _____.
- I am a good mother AND I need <u>a break, to vent, a snack, a nap, time away from my baby</u> (circle one).
- Make up your own!
- Take a picture or a video, or write about those pleasurable/ blissful moments to make them bigger. Imagine you are trying to exaggerate them psychologically and solidify them in your memory.
- Use your hands to exercise your brain.

I recommend to live as if you are traveling in those everyday moments. Imagine you are entering the grocery store for the first time. What do you see, smell, and hear? Engage your senses around you. Is there a new product you never tried? Peruse. Observe. Take it in. Go for a walk and imagine you're exploring a new countryside. What details are new and what can you focus on? What does the pattern on that bird look like? What does that flower smell like? When we are traveling to new places, it's easier for us to immerse ourselves in the novelty. However, there is plenty of novelty in everyday life if you can teach yourself how to look for it.

Now, all this talk about positive emotions may leave you feeling unseen. As countless patients of mine inquire, "What about the actual negative experiences? Am I just supposed to 'choose' to divert my attention during the late-night feedings, lack of sleep, smelly diapers, fussy moments, sick days, boredom, monotony, irritability, spit-ups, meltdowns, food refusal, tantrums, hitting, 'I hate you, Mommy,' throwing objects, sibling fights?" The list can go on and on. There is no shortage of moments that absolutely suck in parenthood. Remember our rule: *do not make it worse*. To me, that means not dwelling, not focusing too much on it, not making it bigger than it needs to be, not starting a fight with my husband about it or including the laundry list of items from prior fights, and not taking the bait when he tries to start one with me.

It helps me to slow things down, to start taking deep breaths and pausing, asking myself, *Will doing this strengthen or weaken a negative neural network in my brain?* If my reaction or focus on the experience does not serve to weaken the network, I will do my best to let it go. Sometimes that means going for a walk; or sticking my head in a bowl of ice cubes; or going line by line in a book, circling every other *a* until the urge to ruminate or rant passes. Sometimes it means just shifting focus and changing the channel in our brains to something else.

How to Self-Direct Maternal Neuroplasticity

- Practice gratitude as an antidote to fear in moments of joy.
- In negative moments, remind yourself of this question: "Do I want to make this negative neural network stronger or weaker?" Remember, *don't make it worse.*
- Give yourself credit! Make mistakes and be compassionate with yourself. Be curious about how that could go differently the next time. As you complete each new task, integrate it within yourself. No task is too small. For example: "My baby had diaper rash. I have been doing a great job applying the diaper cream regularly and comforting my baby. I am proud of myself for all tasks, small and large. It's a lot to keep track of to take care of a baby, and I have never done this before."

Thriving is not the absence of triggers or bad days or challenging moments. Thriving is being able to bring yourself back, let go, and move forward. Remember the upward spiral in motherhood. Thriving is freedom from mental health symptoms interfering with your ability to enjoy life. I am free and I am hoping that, by sharing these stories, I can help you find your freedom. And it is still work to be free even when you are thriving.

Productivity looks different in motherhood. Slowing down, growing a baby inside you, nurturing and growing a mother inside you, taking care of infants and toddlers—these are all extremely productive enterprises. Just keeping a baby alive is an enormous accomplishment. These endeavors take time, lots of time. The pace at which this happens can feel lightning fast and slow as molasses at the same time. I want you to tell yourself you are working to create, reinforce, and guide healthy neural networks in your brain. Oftentimes, this means slowing down reactivity, pausing, breathing, thinking, remaining still, and *not doing.* This looks very different from corporate productivity, or productivity that you may have experienced pre-baby. I want you to hold in your mind that you are serving as a model for how to develop resilience and approach hard things. While you are strengthening your healthy networks, your baby's neural networks are forming interdependent of yours. If you are steady, your baby's networks will be steady.

The phenological plasticity phenomenon refers to brain changes related to interactions with external stimuli. In line with this process that occurs in parenting, Chelsea Conaboy's 2022 book, *Mother Brain*, highlights the research that dispels the notion that maternal instinct is only biological. She summarizes that of course pregnancy, delivery, and lactation give a head start to mothers, but that all primary caregivers are then transformed by the behavioral acts of child-rearing. There has been much research to support a neural caregiver network in which all caregivers involved in intense child-rearing may benefit. In short, the environmental impact of hands-on parenting and caregiving is somewhat less pronounced and very similar to brain changes in mothers.

During the period of becoming a mother, the maternal brain is primed and in the best shape for learning. It is reasonable to conclude the same for fathers and allocaregivers. Hands-on parenting makes you smarter. It forces you to learn, adapt, think creatively, problem-solve, and anticipate needs in a timely, important, and relentless manner. Parents are forced to rise to the challenges of child-rearing, and this ultimately improves their brain functioning.

It is important to take advantage of this opportunity to nurture this development and remove obstacles, including mental health conditions that can occur in all primary caregivers. We should view this developmental phase as an asset, an advantage to families, society, and the workplace. The messaging given to parents should be that your brain can be better than ever if you can nurture and trust this process. Remember, this is an optimal time to integrate other material that can be learned, such as learning how to better care for yourself; learning how to better regulate your own emotions; gaining insight into your own psychological constitution; learning about what type of parent you want to be; learning about your own triggers and how you were mothered and parented; learning about your own needs; learning how to make space for yourself; and learning about how to cultivate creativity, fun, and flexibility in this demanding phase.

SNAPSHOT

How to Self-Direct Maternal Neuroplasticity

- It is your job to protect your brain.
- Thriving is not the absence of triggers, bad days, and challenging moments.
- Remember, productivity looks different in motherhood.
- Brain changes occur in fathers and allocaregivers too, through phenotypic plasticity. The greater their involvement, the greater the neuroplastic changes.
- Maternal instinct is not biological.

Another activity I like to recommend to promote self-directed neuroplasticity is mom flow. Flow is a transcendent state of mind when you are completely immersed in the activity at hand and lose track of time. It is a peak experience that engages you in the present and cultivates productivity, enjoyment, and meaning. Typically, I experience flow when I have consecutive hours to paint, write, or create. Perhaps you have experienced flow in your work, your creative endeavors, cooking, or socializing with friends. Flow can happen anywhere. I love flow. Flow is intoxicating.

After becoming a mom of two, finding consecutive hours to get into flow during writing was simply not possible. As I grieved the loss of those hours, a strange thing began to happen. Previously, I thought flow would not be possible to achieve without an hour or more of open time, so I would not engage in the creative tasks I usually enjoy. But then I realized that was not serving me. So I started to experiment. I began trying to get into the flow state quicker by ignoring the chatter in my mind that said, "But you only have 45 minutes" or "The baby will wake up soon" or "You don't have time for that." I tried. During an hour while my baby napped, a half-hour break while my husband did bath time or tended to both of the little ones, I quickly snuck off and wrote a passage, painted one shade on a canvas, or created one sentence to start an opinion piece. I jumped at any opportunity.

In the beginning, I would get frustrated when the moment was interrupted or over, having really enjoyed being in flow. I quieted that voice too, accepting it and praising myself for getting anything done. Then it happened: I achieved flow in briefer intervals of time. Like strengthening a new muscle, the more I practiced these brief stints of activity, the easier it would be to get into flow faster. Flow is certainly not how it looked pre-baby, but then again, nothing else is either. Instead of chasing what was before, move forward through the process and cultivate your new "mom flow." All is not lost. It is just different. It's waiting for you.

Creativity builds on itself. The opposite of depression is expression. When we are in a stable or positive mood, we are able to think clearly and more creatively, whether it be for problem-solving for creative projects, or negotiating with your toddler to resist jumping off the top of his play kitchen. In this vein, I am reminded of a former patient. Delia was a graphic designer for a corporate company prior to having her first child. She sought out therapy from me because her maternity leave was coming to an end. She was supposed to return to work in three weeks, and because her baby was only nine weeks old, she was having trouble imagining having the capacity to "create" anything during this time. We worked through her transition back to work, and I helped her find processes and conditions to help her "create" again. Mom flow was especially helpful for her.

SNAPSHOT

How to Self-Direct Maternal Neuroplasticity

- Flow is a transcendent state of mind when you are completely immersed in the activity at hand and lose track of time.
- Flow is a peak experience that engages you in the present and cultivates productivity, enjoyment, and meaning.
- Finding consecutive hours to do an activity or work may be challenging in early motherhood.
- Grieve the loss of those consecutive days/hours/weekends that you could spend doing an activity of pleasure and flow.
- It is possible to train your maternal brain to get into the state of flow when you have briefer blocks of time available.

In getting into mom flow or a space of creativity, you can also apply the questions I introduced earlier in this chapter: "Which neural networks do you want to reinforce today?" or, alternatively, "Which neural networks are not serving you, so you can work toward getting rid of them?" (aka synaptic pruning). You can also quiet your thoughts to enter into creative space. Eventually, one small gain leads to the next and the next. That's the thing with cultivating positive emotions and creativity: they build on one another. Each experience builds on the next and broadens one's mindset. That's why it's called the Broaden-and-Build theory of positive emotions in the field of positive psychology. Ultimately, the neural networks around the dead-end negativity fade and become harder to access.

Mom flow means keep saying yes to holding the space to get into flow. Then practice quieting your mind and jumping in to the task at hand. If intrusive thoughts pop up about the baby or to-do lists, say to yourself, "I will think about this after flow time." With practice and over time, you will become better at getting into flow faster, and your flow will become increasingly more productive.

My patients tell me how much it helps them to think of their brain and helping it function better, to have the understanding of what they are working with and how to facilitate the adaptive neural mechanisms while getting rid of the ones that don't serve them. Or, as one patient said after she decided not to go down the rabbit hole worrying about what the other mother thought about her after their children's play date, "I am pruning!" This does not mean you will not experience negativity or negative emotions; it means you won't unnecessarily ruminate, obsess, focus, and make bigger what will not help you.

SNAPSHOT

How to Self-Direct Maternal Neuroplasticity

Follow these steps to get into mom flow:

- Bring yourself into the present and quiet your mind. Let go of distracting thoughts.
- Choose the activity that you've been putting off, preferably a creative outlet (e.g., painting, writing, creating something, reading, rock climbing, playing music, building, designing, card making, singing, playing tennis, baking, crafting).
- Accept that now is not the ideal time to do the activity.
- Start the activity anyway and immerse yourself.
- If you get interrupted or when you have to stop mid-flow, accept the frustration. Don't fight it.
- Name one thing you were grateful for during the activity.
- Repeat all these steps and practice.
- The more you practice, the quicker you will get into mom flow.

12

HOW TO HANDLE TRANSITIONS: BACK TO WORK

"Like a small boat on the ocean. Sending big waves into motion. This is my fight song, take back my life song."
—RACHEL PLATTEN, "FIGHT SONG"

I had two very different experiences returning to work after having children. With my first, my employer generously gave me four months' maternity leave, which I thought would be ample time. But I stalled, and when month five rolled around, I tearfully told her, "I am not ready to come back yet." With two kids now in college, she empathically responded, "I remember that time." I didn't return to the office until Jordan was six months old. Even then, with a trusted nanny at home, the 50-minute commute felt too long. I still didn't feel ready, but with my breast pump bag in hand and pump times scheduled between meetings and patients, I did feel prepared. My first day back, with my hands-free pump bra in place and milking cups intact, I reached into the bag for the final cap to seal the pump in place and found . . . nothing. I had left one of the caps on the counter, probably when I was washing and drying the pieces after the middle-of-the-night pump. That Medela just stared at me from my desk, as dejected and useless as I felt. I had to leave my office early that day to pump at home.

With my second child, I was determined to do things differently. By that time, I had established a full-time private practice. That meant no benefits, such as paid maternity leave. But it didn't matter. My practice meant freedom to me, and I loved my patients. Work was finally in a place where I wanted it—full and a steady flow of referrals. While I was thrilled for Max to arrive, I felt a little disappointed about taking time away from my work. I decided that I would take one month fully off, then slowly increase to one day a week for the second month, two days a week for the third month, and three days a week for the fourth month. I hoped that by five or six months, my practice would be back to where it was prior to me leaving. I was determined to maintain my practice *and* take care of Max.

How do you know when, or if, you are ready to go back to work? You may not ever feel ready. This does not mean that you should not go back to work. It means that readiness occurs after you sort out how the return will go, making adjustments as you go. If we waited until we were ready to do things before we did them, we would not do a lot of things, such as get married, take that new job, go on that date, or have babies. Being "ready" is a misnomer.

I help my patients understand being ready in this way as well. Transitions are tough, and I hear a lot of moms talk to me about the guilt they have not wanting to leave their children. Or the guilt they feel for wanting to go back to work and leave their children. As I mentioned in the mom guilt chapter, it is optimal for your child if you have something else to care about, whether that be a job, a creative outlet, venture, or other responsibility. Beyond what I have already covered, it is also great for your baby to learn that when a parent leaves the house, they come back, every time.

We work together to come up with how to make the transition easier. Usually it involves conversations with an employer or colleagues to gather information about any temporary flexibility, paid leave possibilities, and potential coverage under the Family and Medical Leave

Act (www.dol.gov/agencies/whd/fmla). Some employers may be willing to extend leave time and/or may offer work-from-home options and remote meetings. A lot of this has changed with COVID, and certain benefits to parents in terms of flexibility and childcare with remote work options have become more common. Make sure you check your company's benefits and policies, and your state laws. You may be entitled to more than you think. (You may also wish to consult an employment lawyer who is familiar with the latest legislation and regulations applicable to residents of your state and can tell you how they apply to your situation.)

Other accommodations that can help ease the transition back to work include working part time for a couple of weeks and then going back full time, if available to you; setting boundaries and understanding what you can say "no" to at work; and not taking on extraneous tasks that are not part of your job responsibilities. If you are planning to pump at work, you may be protected by law. The nursing mothers workplace protections under the Fair Labor Standards Act (see www.dol .gov/sites/dolgov/files/WB/media/508_nursing-mothers_05052022 .pdf) requires that certain eligible employees have practical breaks and a private, protected, uninterrupted space that is not a bathroom area in which to pump.

When you do go back to work, it is imperative that you understand you are an asset to the workplace, even when you don't feel like it. A lot of mothers I work with find it empowering to know that they can successfully manage both work and being a mom. Understand that you have a new engine in your car. You are about to take it on the road and hopefully the highway. It may take some time to get to the highway at full speed, but trust in the process. It is adjusting and adapting to working differently. Your brain, thanks to maternal brain plasticity, coupled with the further shaping from on-the-job training provided by your baby, is now evolved and equipped to handle more and to handle responsibilities differently, even though you may not feel like your brain is enhanced. You may have those common feelings of fog-giness, forgetfulness, and preoccupation with your baby at home. The problem is not those experiences; the problem is the interpretation of those experiences.

Many moms feel like they can't function, or are worse at their job when mistakes, lapses in memory, a forgotten response to an email, or a missed task occurs. Try to remember that these are errors that all humans experience, especially when they are stressed, sleep-deprived, and preoccupied. Don't hyperfocus on these instances. Instead, I want to empower moms to understand that their brain functioning is differ-ent, not worse, and in some cases better. We just need to adjust to work-ing differently. Like any change, it takes time to understand exactly how to use these changes to your advantage in your job. Notice if you work better at different hours of the day. Then plan out your job responsi-bilities according to priority, importance, and brain power needed. For example, perhaps you are slow to start in the morning. Maybe when you first arrive and settle in to work, this would be the opportune time to do the more mundane tasks of your job, such as answering emails, scheduling, or organizing your desk. Then, if you find you are most effi-cient later in the morning, try to schedule your meetings or tasks that require the most brain power at those times. Your energy, efficiency, and attention may ebb and flow throughout the day. Observe and try to align your daily work schedule with those times.

In addition, when making "interpretations" about those lapses, mistakes, or interruptions by baby-related needs (daycare calls, baby illness, pumping, etc.), remind yourself that you are just beginning to take your new car out on the road. You know you're working with a souped-up engine underneath, but you still need time and practice to figure out which roads to take, which gas to use, which gear to shift into, what speed, and what music you'll be listening to on the drive. You also have to take into account the metaphorical weather, traffic jams, and construction detours. These blips early on are just detours.

Eventually it will come together better than ever, but being self-critical, quitting, or avoiding the test-drives, will only make the drive worse.

On the other hand, you may find yourself more efficient at work in different ways. You may find yourself saying no to the tasks that are not part of your essential role because you have a newfound appreciation for prioritizing what is important. Or you understand that your resources are limited and you want to be strategic in how you allocate them. I encourage that, especially in the beginning of the return-to-work phase. You are already embarking on some very essential work.

I know this about your brain, and now you do too, and I hope you can keep it in the back of your mind when you are adjusting back to work. I want you to know your value and the value of your maternal brain. Too often employers do not. It saddens me to think of the many ways that mothers are disadvantaged when they return to work. A recent article published on Study Finds includes the challenges that many moms face when going back to work, such as lack of self-confidence, missed opportunities for promotion, biases and negative judgments about work commitment, and lack of support from employers and colleagues.[36]

The maternal brain is often mentioned in the same breath as a series of perceived shortcomings, lapses, and subjective memory loss. But remember, Jodi Pawluski's recent article explains that numerous studies show a lack of strong evidence of memory deficits, despite mothers' subjective experience of feeling "foggy" or forgetful.

To review, research extends beyond the minimal losses and points to the cognitive enhancements experienced through maternal brain plasticity. In several studies, it was shown pregnant women actually experienced "boosts in learning" on baby-related tasks and had better long-term memory overall compared to nonpregnant women.[37] Other maternal brain studies show mothers are better at "mentalizing" and social intelligence,[38] and, over time, mothers continue to improve their skills in caregiving, understanding emotional experiences, and parental vigilance.[39] Another study showed that mothers, compared to non-mothers, scored higher on brain activity associated with social cognition, including theory of mind and empathy, and demonstrated increased cognitive efficiency and a "more responsive, flexible, and efficient emotion-regulation system."[40] In a recent study examining the benefits of motherhood, it was stated that many qualities that emerge from motherhood, such as emotional intelligence, motivation, and capacity for knowledge, are desirable in the workplace.

The time has come for mothers to know their worth in the workplace and to acknowledge the brilliance of the maternal brain—both tremendous assets to employers, companies, and clients. Mothers are at a unique advantage when they go through matrescence, the single greatest period of neuroplasticity in the briefest period of time. These significant brain changes, coupled with the "mental load" of motherhood, force mothers to adapt immensely to their heightened responsibilities, but they are faced with incredible challenges during an opportune time to learn. Their brain continues to fine-tune itself while rising to each new challenge, and as a result, they have the potential to increase cognitive reserve in the long term. Mothers can reach their full potential as long as they are supported by solid mental health treatment, stress management during postpartum, fair division of labor at home, and opportunities to nurture the psychological processes of neuroplasticity and post-traumatic growth.[41]

We have an opportunity to better support mothers in their return to work and to engage them in their work. When the plasticity process goes right, it can go really right. In time, what can emerge is a smarter, more efficient, creative, and productive employee. No one is a better problem-solver and more efficient than a mother who has to soothe, feed, play, engage, bond, clean, and tend to all the needs on demand from an infant. The maternal brain supports this adaptation, and the skill set can translate to the office. Let's empower mothers to understand what they are working with under the hood and educate employers to better understand their mistakenly undertapped resource.

In fact, I am so impassioned by the potential of the maternal brain, I drafted a letter for mothers going back to work to imagine sending to their employers.

Dear Employer:

As I prepare to return to work on _____[date], I wanted to update you and the team on my reintegration. As you may already know, I gave birth to a healthy baby boy/girl on [XX/XX/XXXX] named _____. I have been fortunate to have this time to take care of him/her and welcome the opportunity to introduce additional responsibilities back into my life.

This early phase of mothering has been transformative in so many ways, including biologically. While I may look the same, the cells underneath are different from those I had before giving birth. My hair color is the same, but it covers something very different underneath, an expanded and evolved maternal brain that is more efficient, fine-tuned, and better equipped than ever before. My increased brain power is facilitating my ability to rise to a vicissitude of challenges. I welcome new opportunities to continue to demonstrate my capabilities.

Before I left, I know there was discussion about a [project, promotion, client, opportunity] that was coming up, and I am eager to hear more about the current status and think together about how I can use my newly gained assets to enhance this [said project/promotion/client/opportunity]. In these early days of parenting, I have risen to the relentless challenges a newborn begs and have come out the other side. I am proud of myself for my efforts and have also learned a great deal that will influence my work for the better. I have a better understanding of what is essential and how to complete work efficiently (no doubt the result of the around-the-clock schedule of feeding, cleaning, nurturing, stimulating, and tending to my own needs), all of which I have done and continue to do successfully.

Now for the most important part. You have the unique opportunity to benefit from my new role as a mother. My brain is in the early phase of postpartum maternal plasticity. In other words, hormones, neurotransmitters, and structural and functional changes are occurring as we speak to help me better tend to my child's needs. In addition, with the help of science, I have been integrating unique strategies to better tend to my needs, so I can thrive during this intense phase of caregiving.

I invite you to take part in the opportunity to benefit from these neuroplastic changes and to allow our work together to benefit. I would love to discuss how we can support this process together. I encourage you to approach me with new projects and ideas you may otherwise feel hesitant to put on the plate of a new mother. I would love to review any and all ideas together to see what would most benefit from my enhanced brain power. I may not be able to say yes to every new opportunity, but I promise to work with you to determine which projects would benefit most from my concentrated efforts. While I am more efficient than ever before, I also want us to focus on what is most essential for our incredible team, company, project, etc. and myself.

I look forward to enhancing our workplace soon with my mom brain.

Sincerely yours,
Me

This letter is not necessarily meant for you to send to your employer; it is for you to keep in mind as you are adjusting to being back at work. The letter puts the emphasis on the many advantages you offer to your work environment, which you should keep in mind on days when you forget your breast pump part. Or are low energy from another sleepless night. Or completed that presentation but are harping on that one missed point that came to you later in the day. Or are embarrassed by that awkward interaction with a colleague because your breasts were leaking. Or realized you forgot to tell the babysitter where your baby's pacifier is and had to run to make a phone call. Or when you are killing it during a new client meeting, only to be interrupted by daycare because your baby spiked a fever. It's these words I want you to hold on to when you are dressed and ready to get out the door on time, but then your baby projectile vomits onto your only unwrinkled outfit. It's the work happy hour you can no longer attend or lunch with the high-powered executives you have to skip because you need to pump. I want to help you understand how you are, and will continue to be, an asset to any venture. Remember, in time your brilliant brain is going to thrive at work!

Instead of furthering the uninteresting, inaccurate representation of a mommy brain moment, let's empower mothers to better understand and promote the complicated virtuosity that is the maternal brain. Everyone can benefit from riding this wave of neuroplasticity in motherhood, whether at a place of employment or in the home, raising the future minds of America. The mom mind is resilient—research attests to this. It's also time to flip the script and recognize that mommy brains, even after the pandemic, may in fact be even more evolved than before.

The pandemic was a global trauma.

Pandemic moms have even more to grapple with: they must weigh and consider vaccination status, disease transmission, mental health needs, financial needs, and practical barriers to childcare, and reconfigure the way they function on a daily and evolving basis depending on the variant timeline at play.

The pile-on for moms doesn't stop there. Limited flexible employment options, lack of paid maternity leave, and limited choices for childcare have upped the challenges. Dr. Pooja Lakshmin calls it betrayal, and I agree.[42] Mothers are so stressed out they are being pushed to the brink of screaming.[43] Books such as *I Love You But I've Chosen Darkness*, *The Lost Daughter*, and *Mommy Is Going Away for a While* illustrate that the neural and emotional transition to motherhood is not an easy one, especially now.

Moms need help.

Part of self-care during motherhood is figuring out the work-life balance: when and how to return to work or the decision to stay at home. This choice should not be taken lightly. When determining what the caregiver role for you will look like, there are many factors to consider. Eve Rodsky's *Fair Play* describes the cost of having mothers at home, taking care of children full time. Rodsky maintains that returning to work should not simply be equated with the mother's potential income. In other words, it's not a direct substitution in which mother's income balances daycare cost. Instead, she advocates for the father's or partner's salary to be included in the income bracket because fathers may also benefit from a mother's return to work.

I hear this mental equation all the time from my patients: "It doesn't make sense for me to go back to work," or "It's a wash, so we decided that I should stay home." One particular patient, Emma, recently told me this through tears. Resentment was building up in her marriage. She was with her baby and toddler around the clock, and because she wasn't working, she assumed the majority of the child and household tasks. Emma felt like she could not ask her husband to do more than what he was already doing because this is what they agreed to. The arrangement that easily worked when her first child was in infancy was no longer working as the child entered a new developmental phase and she was now caring for a new baby. She found the particular hands-on parenting to a baby and an older toddler overwhelming.

I asked her, "Okay so how is this working for you now?" Emma suffered from high-functioning depression and anxiety. She was able to take care of her children, but she was struggling with resentment and anger, feeling overwhelmed and panicky. Plus, it was impacting marital satisfaction, which is already at a nadir in general during this early childhood phase. Those effects have no "monetary" value but are extremely costly and must be factored into the decision whether to return to work.

On the flip side, I recently worked with a married, high-powered executive, Peter, whose wife financially did not need to work. He frequently discussed how she would get mad at him if he was late to come home or if he did not help with household tasks. He felt like he was helping and confided in me that he was not sure "what she did all day." Before they were married, she'd agreed to stay home and take care of the kids. He didn't understand why she got angry with him at a sudden change in schedule or why she always seemed to be in a bad mood.

Clinically, this was an opportunity to educate Peter on what high-functioning depression and anxiety may look like. His wife was not my patient, so I could not diagnose her, but I posed the idea that perhaps something more was going on underneath, even when the kids were taken care of and, in his estimation, she had "no reason" to be depressed or anxious. This is often the case in high-functioning depression and anxiety, where the person who is suffering is getting through the day, able to perform tasks at work and at home, and there is no obvious reason that something is off. However, underneath, a clinician can assess for distorted thinking, perfectionistic tendencies, more subtle symptoms of anxiety and depression, and how it is interfering with their ability to enjoy life and get pleasure.

It was also imperative that I work with Peter on his flexibility. Just because this was their prior "agreement" doesn't mean that it is working now. I encourage patients and couples to be flexible throughout the early childhood years, have many discussions, and be prepared to adjust any agreements or arrangements at any time. We have to be open to the possibility that what we thought we wanted may not work for us. It's okay to reassess, renegotiate, and reorganize because there are so many moving parts in early parenthood. Things are always shifting. I advised Peter to have more discussions with his wife about the division of labor and to use the Fair Play card deck to renegotiate responsibilities. Also, it would be helpful for him to understand more about the tasks that seem invisible that his wife is doing and to challenge his distortion "I don't know what she does all day."

When making the decision to go back to work, the arithmetic needs to change. Couples need to consider the psychological cost and benefits in addition to the practical cost and benefits. Furthermore, couples need to be flexible about reassessing how the arrangement is working for them at different times. Remember that division of labor is nuanced and there is no one-size-fits-all approach.

SNAPSHOT

How to Handle Transitions: Back to Work

When making the decision whether to go back to work, the decision should include psychological factors, not simply arithmetic (e.g., maternal income – daycare cost = decision for mother to stay home). The decision to return to work should include:

- Psychological benefit of being engaged in work
- Psychological break from child-rearing
- Contribution to household/finances
- Return-to-work mood benefits on marriage, partnership, and children

13

UP THE ANTE

"All of my best decisions in life have come because I was attuned to what really felt like the next right move for me."
—OPRAH WINFREY

Taking into consideration everything we have covered thus far, I like to think of maternal experiences as opportunities to up the ante. Upping the ante means that, by tending to your own needs first and identifying and managing your own emotions, you fill your cup and expand your bandwidth. This allows you to more easily access your strengths, wisdom, strategies, emotional regulation, patience, and presence to bring forth all your resources to make better decisions. Upping the ante allows you to go a step further and challenge yourself. It can mean anything from doing that relaxation exercise for 30 seconds longer than you think you can or taking on a new creative project or assignment at work. It can mean taking your baby to a grocery store or on an errand you've been avoiding, or going to that new mommy-and-me class. It's making good mothering choices by accessing your resources, deducing from the information you have at the time, and moving in a healthier and more resilient direction. To illustrate, I want to share another personal story with you.

During a recent holiday break, I decided to take up poker. My husband and I were staying at my parents' place with my brothers and their families. Making the most of a full house, my two younger brothers, my sister-in-law, my mom, father, and husband would gather around the dining room table, ready for a respite after long days of caring for our little ones. After bedtime, with our piles of makeshift sunflower seeds as chips, we would gather and place our bets. The two-card, Texas Hold'em game was led by my father, a longtime expert poker player, who taught us how to play.

Over the years, I had picked up pointers from him here and there and was generally familiar with poker, but no doubt, I was a beginner. I respected poker because it's one of the only games where the house does not have an advantage over you. Unless you count my will to win the Mega Millions on my birthday, I have never been much of gambler. You would think after a long day of wrestling with the kids and feeding them their 80th bag of fruit snacks and goldfish, I would sneak off to do something more mindless, like scrolling memes of *The Real Housewives of New York City*, watching *Workin' Moms* on Netflix, or just lying in a dark, silent room. But on days where there was certainly no shortage of stimulation, I was drawn to the table to exercise my mind.

Throughout our friendly family rounds, I learned to fold my cards and "not to fall in love with my hand," as my father would say as I drew a seven-eight suit, trying to pull for a flush. I practiced patience, bluffed sparingly, played good hands, and lost, but the temptation of a new challenge had piqued my interest. The second night, I walked away with the pot.

When I returned home, I had an upcoming trip to Atlantic City planned for a friend's birthday. I decided to prepare by doing a little research. I remembered a quote my brother said at the table as he praised Annie Duke's lessons in the seven-card game: "Learning from outcomes in a haphazard process." I immediately downloaded *Decide to Play Great Poker* and devoured it. Duke's book is dense with knowledge and strategy, but I was excited to learn that, when it comes to poker, there are endless possibilities. Remember, Duke is a former professional poker player and author in cognitive-behavioral decision science and education.

As I read the book, it became clear that the decision process is much like how we make decisions in early motherhood. No two games are the same, and unique factors influence each person, including every outcome and their dynamic within the table. In sum, there is an exponential number of variables to consider when playing. Duke explains that money is just an aside in poker. The true currency is good decision-making. If you base your worth on the outcome, you're missing the point. Duke acknowledges the plethora of books and formulaic strategies that tell you exactly which hands to play and specific algorithms to follow in the game. Similarly, mothers can get stuck on fixed mindsets around breastfeeding, birth plans, sleep schedules, and baby products. Rigidity to ideals is not Duke's game. That is not my game. I recommend that not be your game either.

Both motherhood and poker involve making decisions and taking risks, as well as having to adapt to constantly changing circumstances. Mothers must make decisions about the care of their baby and be able to adapt to the influx of variables that are introduced at any given time. Duke introduces the first two skills in terms of "position" and how to enter the pot with knowledge of your initial two-card hand. Sure, you can focus on rigid rules and methods based on ideals—the perfect baby products, schedule, activities, clothes, which feeding method is best, etc. But becoming a mother and this specific developmental phase offer so much more to consider.

Maternal brain changes; maternal mental health; emotional states, such as mom rage, shame, and guilt; baby bonding; creativity; and identity transition all influence the day-to-day nuts and bolts in early motherhood decision-making. Some days, you are entering the situation navigating several of these factors and some days just one. By taking inventory of our biopsychosocial state, we can have a much more nuanced way of entering each interaction and experience in motherhood. It's not unlike considering the factors important in poker, such as position and how to navigate each turn.

In addition, players must make decisions about which cards to play and be able to adapt to the changing dynamics of the game and their opponents. In poker, Duke instructs you to use "tools, not rules." That is my mission here. Through the information given, I want mothers to shift their understanding about currency in motherhood: good decisions, not outcomes. In this way, even when you lose the battle in the moment, you are winning the war because you are incorporating more knowledge and skills to enhance your decision-making.

When I speak about position in motherhood, it is helpful to understand what state you are in. Your position can change moment to moment, day to day, month to month. For example, if you are struggling with postpartum depression, you are likely going to have trouble experiencing pleasure with your baby and feeling motivated to take on the monotony of the daily routine in infancy. You may be short-fused and shut down, or you might yell when your baby refuses to nap. A mother who is depressed may have less in the tank, get angry, or figure out how to problem-solve. Here, treating maternal depression would take priority. If you are depressed, that will color how you interpret things beyond your baby—a comment by your partner such as "Why don't you sleep when the baby sleeps?"; an encounter with a friend that leaves you feeling embarrassed you are running errands in your maternity clothes; or a male colleague saying, "Oops, there's that mommy brain" when an email goes unanswered.

Feeling depressed can impact your reactivity and can send you into deeper depression. Treating the depression first clears up the picture.

Then, as you move to higher-order constructs, you will be clearer and able to benefit from those challenges. If you are depressed, you are not ready for mom flow. But after treatment, you will be ready to take on and benefit from that transcendent experience.

When thinking about position, I am reminded of Nadia, a patient I recently treated. Nadia reported that she experienced a traumatic birth with her firstborn and was increasingly resentful of her husband (despite his improvements in his own therapy) while she was struggling with "this new life," losing herself, and her own anxiety. She stated that they went to couples therapy regularly but that she feels lost and alone in those sessions and afraid to admit how much she is suffering. When I asked her if she ever sought individual treatment for herself in years prior, when her severe symptoms of anxiety and trauma started, she said no. I found that striking considering she was crying throughout the intake, "What about me?"

I advised her to stop couples therapy and to engage in individual treatment for her symptoms and focus on her own needs. Couples therapy would not work if she was struggling at deeper levels. She reported that couples therapy helped them renegotiate division of labor and communicate about their issues, and also helped her husband be more hands-on in parenting. However, these topics are higher-order constructs. When I think about position for this patient, she needs her clinical symptoms treated before she would benefit from more practical skills, and her depression may be influencing her perception of how she relates to her husband. It is no doubt that all these factors are important, and you also can't do everything all at once. You can't benefit from the higher-order constructs when you don't have the more fundamental mental health intact. This is what I mean by position.

If you are further along, perhaps you are struggling with high-functioning anxiety or healing your mother wound. It is best to tend to those needs first, then tackle more creative higher-order constructs. Perhaps you are triggered by not knowing how to engage your baby with play and giggles. You reflect on your own childhood and recall that you were not allowed to be silly, playful, and loud. Here, would it make more sense to find a surrogate activity to aid with being playful, perhaps a book with sounds, a mommy-and-me music class, a trip to the playground to see other moms engaging their babies, or a television show that provides guidance for "play" with your infant? Or, are you feeling triggered because you need a break and it would help to have a mother's helper or babysitter to delegate play to them? Or perhaps it would be helpful to work through the conflict in therapy and try doing the opposite of what you weren't allowed to do in childhood with your own baby? The truth is, perhaps all of the above at any given time.

Hindsight is 20/20, and you don't have that gift. In the beginning of poker, all you have are your two cards facing you, and the only decision you have is whether to play. The information you use to make this decision is based on position and two cards. When mothering, in each moment, you are given a face value and the position parent with little information. Your maternal brain quickly tries to deduce the issue with the cues in the moment. Sometimes, when you are running on a full night's sleep, a good day at work, or a smooth morning routine with the baby, you're holding an ace king suited. You are present, engaged, rolling with resistance, and problem-solving on the fly. The baby gets to his morning nap without screaming and holding on to you by the crib. The dealer flops three of the same suit, and that's called a flush, my friends—a very good hand.

Each time you make a better decision—more informed, more nuanced, more integrated—you are building and reinforcing adaptive neural networks in your brain. You are making a choice not to go down old, maladaptive, negative neural networks that worsen your mood, limit your options, and make you more rigid. Over time, those less-reinforced neural networks fall away through the process of synaptic pruning. If you don't use it, you will lose it—in a good way. Good riddance! Out with the old and in with the new.

Even better news: these new neural networks expand and strengthen over time and become easier to access. In other words, the more you practice these strategies and reinforce the helpful neural networks in your brain, the easier it will be to take those roads. Eventually they will run like highway express lanes. By broadening and building your repertoire of skills, you have the opportunity to become even better than before. You can nurture your brain and continue to challenge it to go further.

Maybe the next time your baby is crying you can be patient for 30 seconds longer. That gives you 30 more seconds to problem-solve, contain emotions, and delay reactivity. Congratulations. You have just improved your resiliency. The next time, that 30 seconds will be easier because you have done it before, learned what it takes to stay in that time, and problem-solved more effectively. Then you get to a minute, five minutes, and so on. Then you find yourself less triggered overall and knowing how to pull yourself out of episodes of mom rage, guilt, and shame more quickly. This in turn weakens harmful neural networks, and the process continues. I can't promise that you will not be triggered again, endure mental health crises, or experience being overstimulated, touched out, rageful, depressed, or anxious. You are human and a mother. Feelings are fleeting. This will pass. Remember, change and development are not linear. So we expect these "relapses." You do, however, come to those similar feelings, dilemmas, challenges, and experiences with stronger maternal brain development and more strategies to make even better, more informed decisions.

Perhaps you are wondering what happened when I took my newly enhanced mommy brain to the actual poker table. I was riding high with residual hubris from my wins at my family's house and signed myself up for a seat at the table. I craved more challenges since becoming a mother. The truth is, the other players sized me up as soon as I walked through the door. It was clear I was no longer playing for sunflower seeds; I lost all my money in 10 minutes. But, here's the good news: I am not teaching you how to play poker.

My decision-making abilities improved by pressing me to learn quickly, even if I lost. Poker involves a lot of complex brain power and forces you to make decisions quickly, in real time, and much faster than playing with my family. I went into it with low expectations and low budget. Good decisions were the currency and money was not the outcome. I knew the margaritas would work against me (again taking position into account). It was my goal to see if I had to play tight or could loosen a bit and deduce if I had a playable hand. Then I entered the pot raising the blind, testing what I had learned in Duke's first chapters, each move building new neural systems in my brain.

I imagined that, since I had never played in a live poker match at a casino, my neural networks had not been formed. I actually pictured what a nugget of a newly created neural network would look like in my brain. I imagined a seedling of a plant just peeking through soil. This visualization put things in perspective about what it takes to induce neuroplasticity. I was trying to build neural networks in real time, little by little, in 10 minutes of decision-making. I finished my hands and look forward to reinforcing those networks in another game, perhaps something more like canasta.

Until then, I'll continue upping the ante—pausing before I react to my mom guilt, shame, and rage; tending to my needs to make a deliberate decision; saying yes to something just outside my comfort zone; finding ways to practice mom flow; being assertive in division of labor; taking on creative challenges; and broadening and building my own resiliency. Motherhood is my motivation to continue to up the ante in my life, having brought with it a renewed sense of purpose and meaning. I will continue to thrive and play each hand better than the last, even when I hit a patch of panic about Max ingesting a foreign object, or the rotating stomach bug at daycare, or the guilt that pits in my stomach when I choose that girls dinner over bedtime, or the next time I want to rage at my husband for forgetting to pack the swim diapers. I encourage you to do the same.

So go ahead and take your new extraordinary mommy brain out for a spin and enjoy feeling less rattled.

Top Ten Tips

1. When you become a mother, the brain goes through major neuroplastic changes that can work for and against you. Nurture the process and protect your brain.
2. Set up a postpartum mental health care plan with a pre-scriber and a licensed mental health professional whether you think you will need them or not. Schedule follow-up visits within two weeks post-birth and then follow up regularly. You may also coincide your appointments with changes in breastfeeding/nursing.
3. Heal your mother wound if you have one. Grieve the mother you never had or the needs that weren't met when you were a child. Channel that energy into meeting those needs of your baby.
4. Remember the golden rule in motherhood: self-care is not selfish. You cannot serve from an empty vessel.
5. Baby bonding typically takes months. Be patient with yourself and the process.
6. Double down on mom guilt. Perhaps the thing that makes you feel guilty is the thing you need to be doing.
7. Soften on mom shame. Tend compassionately to that wounded girl inside you. How can you comfort her?
8. When you experience mom rage, *don't make it worse*. Tend to your triggered feelings first.
9. Use techniques to self-direct the maternal neuroplastic changes that occur during this powerful phase of motherhood.
10. Challenge yourself to up the ante in motherhood. Your brain will continue to fine-tune and develop further resiliency the more you can engage in more challenging activities. You can be better than ever.

ACKNOWLEDGMENTS

Gratitude, we know, is a positive emotion. It serves to broaden our mindsets and fosters resiliency by allowing us to build more adaptive neural networks. Expressing gratitude every day makes us happier.

I know this to be true. All along the journey of researching, writing, and producing *Rattled*, I have been amazed, grateful, and, yes, joyful because of the many people who have supported me. Thank you to my agent, Marilyn Allen, for believing in the power of the book from the start. Thank you for always advocating for my best interests and for astute guidance. Thank you to my editor, Ann Treistman, for her impactful feedback that helped cultivate this book: part science, part art, and, most importantly, the story I always wanted to tell. Her edits have guided me and ensured only the best components made it into this book. I am grateful for her responsiveness, respect, and openness.

Thank you to my marketing team, Devorah Backman and Zachary Polendo, for distilling the essence of this book into concise marketing materials and for promoting *Rattled* to various media in advance of the book's release. I appreciate both of your efforts behind the scenes.

Thank you to Maya Goldfarb and the rest of my team at Countryman Press for getting *Rattled* out in an efficient, powerful, and aesthetically pleasing way.

I have been fortunate to work with incredible mentors and teams throughout my professional career that have no doubt influenced my thinking and creativity, each of whom contributed to my writing *Rattled*. First and foremost, I want to thank my psychotherapist and thought partner, Dr. Frank. Words on this page cannot do justice to how much you have helped me in every facet of my modern life. Your brilliant, thought-provoking, uncanny insight have facilitated my growth as a human, a mother, a wife, daughter, sister, friend, and most recently, a writer.

The journey to becoming a licensed clinical psychologist is arduous and challenging and requires significant guidance, mentorship, and encouragement. I have been fortunate to work with the best of the best and it would be impossible to name the countless professionals that have shaped my life. Know that I am grateful for the big and small gestures that have supported me along the way.

I'm grateful to my community at the University of Rhode Island for providing exceptional doctoral training in Clinical Psychology. Special thanks to Dr. Mark Robbins, Dr. Andrea Paiva, the late Dr. James Prochaska, Dr. Colleen Redding, and Dr. Ellen Flannery Schroeder for being sources of positivity and support.

To Dr. Joseph Greer from Harvard Medical School and the Massachusetts General Hospital, for his mentorship, compassionate wisdom, and guidance, thank you. To Dr. Jean Kutner, for taking me on as an NIH-T32 Fellow in Aging and Palliative Care at the University of Colorado Anschutz Medical Campus, thank you. To the late Dr. Mark Laudenslager, for introducing me to caregiver research and the importance of their needs, thank you. Your support in Pep-Pal was instrumental in improving resources for caregivers.

Thanks go to a host of leading maternal researchers and writers whose expertise and discussions on this book were crucial for the production of *Rattled*: Katherine Ellison, Katherine Lambert, PhD; Elseline Hoekzema, PhD; Pilyoung Kim, PhD; Jodi Pawluski, PhD; Jessica Vernon, MD; Helena Rutherford, PhD; and Bridget Callaghan, PhD. To Eve Rodsky, for her generosity of time, support, and endorsement of *Rattled*. To Zibby Owens, for publishing my first editorial on postpartum mental health and support for *Rattled*. To Sarah Alter, a true mompreneur. To Adam Alter, for taking the time between writing best-selling novels to provide his endorsement for *Rattled*. To Rick Hanson, PhD, for his work on neural plasticity that inspired segments of this book and for endorsing this publication. To Spencer, for early brainstorming meetings. To Gina Hamadey, for her initial meeting about this book proposal.

To all of my patients that I feel privileged to work with, I give my heartfelt thanks to the mothers and daughters that have inspired compilations in this book; thank you for allowing me to care for you.

I am indebted to my mom village, for their encouragement and support. Thank you to Dr. Elizabeth Reichert and Dr. Jamie Jacobs, for endorsing *Rattled*. To my best friends that are my sisters, thank you for listening to run-throughs, excerpts, and ideas for *Rattled*. You know who you are, especially Brooke, Stacey, and Heather.

This entire book is about the help that all mothers need. I am the beneficiary of an enormously loving and close family, and this book could not be here without their support. It is through their loving support that I am able to build my own family and reflect on that process. Their love is the backbone of the book.

To my mother and father, who are role models for helping others. To my mother, for loving me and breaking cycles; for always seeing my strengths and for reminding me of them; for having high expectations and never letting me sell myself short when it truly mattered. I cherish our conversations about motherhood because they have brought us closer, and for all that you have sacrificed. To my father, whose work ethic and selflessness is unparalleled, for always putting other people first and serving as my role model for empathizing with others; for his entrepreneurial wisdom, reassuring fatherly insight, and steadfast guidance are my beacons in life.

To my brothers, Tony and Joseph, who are both sources of great strength and endless laughter and whose collective creativity is inspiring. To my sister-in-law, Hillary, for her sharp marketing eye and raising kids side-by-side with me. To my beloved in-laws, Sandy and Alan, for their unconditional love, and to my sister-in-law, Robyn, and her husband Alan, to my cousin Roni for his early support for the book, and the rest of my extended family.

To my children. My daughter, Jordan, who listens so deeply, offers insights and suggestions, and cares so much about the world. I love you and give thanks for you. My son, Max, who floods every moment with enjoyment and curiosity, the kindest and playful soul that delights everyone around you. Jordan and Max, being your mother is the single greatest joy in my life. You amaze me nothing less than every single day. I love you always and give thanks for you.

Last here, but first in my life, to Mike, for the generous and honest content, late night edits, run-throughs, foot massages, and making me laugh; for being my rock in the trenches; for being the best daddy to our little ones; and for being my soul mate and partner in this beautiful and complicated life. None of this is possible without you.

NOTES

1. Barba-Müller, E., Craddock, S., Carmona, S., & Hoekzema, E. (2019). Brain plasticity in pregnancy and the postpartum period: links to maternal caregiving and mental health. *Archives of Women's Mental Health*, 22, 289–299. https://doi.org/10.1007/s00737-018-0889-z

2. Pawluski, J. L., Hoekzema, E., Leuner, B., & Lonstein, J. S. (2022). Less can be more: Fine tuning the maternal brain. *Neuroscience & Biobehavioral Reviews*, 133, 104475. https://doi.org/10.1016/j.neubiorev.2021.11.045

3. Abu-Raya, B., Michalski, C., Sadarangani, M., & Lavoie, P. M. (2020). Maternal immunological adaptation during normal pregnancy. *Frontiers in Immunology*, 11. https://doi.org/10.3389/fimmu.2020.575197

4. Barrett, J., Wonch, K. E., Gonzalez, A., Ali, N., Steiner, M., Hall, G. B., & Fleming, A. S. (2012). Maternal affect and quality of parenting experiences are related to amygdala response to infant faces. *Social Neuroscience*, 7(3), 252–268. https://doi.org/10.1080/17470919.2011.609907

5. Barba-Müller, E., et al. (2019). Brain plasticity in pregnancy and the postpartum period: Links to maternal caregiving and mental health, 289–299.

6. Centers for Disease Control and Prevention. (n.d.). *Depression among women*. https://www.cdc.gov/reproductivehealth/depression/index.htm

7. Mateus, V., Cruz, S., Costa, R., Mesquita, A., Christoforou, A., Wilson, C. A., Vousoura, E., Dikmen-Yildiz, P., Bina, R., Dominguez-Salas, S., Contreras-García, Y., Motrico, E., & Osório, A. (2022). Rates of depressive and anxiety symptoms in the perinatal period during the COVID-19 pandemic: Comparisons between countries and with pre-pandemic data.

Journal of Affective Disorders, 316, 245–253. https://doi.org/10.1016/j.jad .2022.08.017

8. Arnold, M., & Kalibatseva, Z. (2021). Are "Superwomen" without social support at risk for postpartum depression and anxiety? *Women & Health*, 61(2), 148–159. https://doi.org/10.1080/03630242.2020.1844360

9. Huller Harari, L., Blasbalg, U., Arnon, S., Ben-Sheetrit, J., & Toren, P. (2022). Risk factors for postpartum depression among sexual minority and heterosexual parents. *Australasian Psychiatry: Bulletin of Royal Australian and New Zealand College of Psychiatrists*, 30(6), 718–721. https://doi.org/10 .1177/10398562221133990

10. Barba-Müller, E., et al. (2019). Brain plasticity in pregnancy and the postpartum period: Links to maternal caregiving and mental health, 289–299.

11. Kim, P. (2016). Human maternal brain plasticity: Adaptation to parenting. *New Directions for Child and Adolescent Development*, 2016(153), 47–58. https://doi.org/10.1002/cad.20168

12. Orchard, E. R., Voigt, K., Chopra, S., Thapa, T., Ward, P. G. D., Egan, G. F., & Jamadar, S. D. (2023). The maternal brain is more flexible and responsive at rest: Effective connectivity of the parental caregiving network in postpartum mothers. *Scientific Reports*, 13, 4719. https://doi.org/10.1038/ s41598-023-31696-4

13. Kolb, B., & Muhammad, A. (2014). Harnessing the power of neuroplasticity for intervention. *Frontiers in Human Neuroscience*, 8. https://doi.org/10 .3389/fnhum.2014.00377

14. Miller, V., & Price-Crist, M. (2023). Mommy brain in the United States. *Ethos*, 51, 111–129. https://doi.org/10.1111/etho.12381

15. McCormack, C., Callaghan, B. L., & Pawluski, J. L. (2023). It's time to rebrand "mommy brain." *JAMA Neurology*, 80(4), 335–336. https://doi .org/10.1001/jamaneurol.2022.5180

16. Orchard, E. R., et al. (2023). The maternal brain is more flexible and responsive at rest: Effective connectivity of the parental caregiving network in postpartum mothers, 4719.

17. Orchard, E. R., Rutherford, H. J. V., Holmes, A. J., & Jamadar, S. D. (2023). Matrescence: Lifetime impact of motherhood on cognition and the brain. *Trends in Cognitive Science*, 27(3), 302–316. https://doi.org/10.1016/j .tics.2022.12.002

18. Wu, X., Kaminga, A. C., Dai, W., Deng, J., Wang, Z., Pan, X., & Liu, A. (2019). The prevalence of moderate-to-high posttraumatic growth: A systematic review and meta-analysis. *Journal of Affective Disorders*, 243, 408–415. https://doi.org/10.1016/j.jad.2018.09.023

19. Pawluski, J. L., et al. (2022). Less can be more: Fine tuning the maternal brain, 104475.

20. Hoekzema, E., van Steenbergen, H., Straathof, M., Beekmans, A., Freund, I. M., Pouwels, P. J. W., & Crone, E. A. (2022). Mapping the

effects of pregnancy on resting state brain activity, white matter micro-structure, neural metabolite concentrations and grey matter archi-tecture. *Nature Communications*, 13, 6931. https://doi.org/10.1038/s41467-022-33884-8

21. Feldman, R., Braun, K., & Champagne, F. A. (2019). The neural mechanisms and consequences of paternal caregiving. *Nature Reviews Neuroscience*, 20, 205–224. https://doi.org/10.1038/s41583-019-0124-6

22. Kotelchuck, M. (2022). The impact of fatherhood on men's health and development. In Grau Grau, M., las Heras Maestro, M., & Riley Bowles, H. (eds.), *Engaged Fatherhood for Men, Families and Gender Equality. Contributions to Management Science*, 63–91. Springer, Cham. https://doi.org/10.1007/978-3-030-75645-1_4

23. Chung, G. (2023, March 24). Hayden Panettiere shares what really "hurts" about postpartum struggles. *E! News*. https://www.eonline.com/news/1369252/hayden-panettiere-shares-what-really-hurts-about-postpartum-struggles

24. Fairbrother, N., Collardeau, F., Albert, A. Y. K., Challacombe, F. L., Thordarson, D. S., Woody, S. R., & Janssen, P. A. (2021). High preva-lence and incidence of obsessive-compulsive disorder among women across pregnancy and the postpartum. *The Journal of Clinical Psychiatry*, 82(2), 20m13398. https://doi.org/10.4088/JCP.20m13398

25. Sacks, A. (2017, May 8). The birth of a mother. *The New York Times*. https://www.nytimes.com/2017/05/08/well/family/the-birth-of-a-mother.html

26. Harvard Health Publishing. (2012, August 30). Feeling down? It could be low-level depression. *Healthbeat*, Harvard Medical School. https://www.health.harvard.edu/healthbeat/feeling-down-it-could-be-low-level-depression

27. Delva, S. (2016, September 14). The Signs of High-Functioning Depression. *Orchid Recovery Center Blog*. https://www.orchidrecoverycenter.com/blog/the-signs-of-high-functioning-depression

28. Alkon, C. (n.d.). *Treating sexual problems: An interview with Virginia Sadock, MD*. Western New York Urology Associates. https://www.wnyurology.com/content.aspx?chunkiid=14493

29. Constantinou, G., Varela, S., & Buckby, B. (2021). Reviewing the expe-riences of maternal guilt—The "motherhood myth" influence. *Health Care for Women International*, 42(4–6), 852–876. https://doi.org/10.1080/07399332.2020.1835917

30. Gould, N. F., McKibben, J. B., Hall, R., Corry, N. H., Amoyal, N. A., Mason, S. T., McCann, U. D., & Fauerbach, J. A. (2011). Peritraumatic heart rate and posttraumatic stress disorder in patients with severe burns. *The Journal of Clinical Psychiatry*, 72(4), 539–547. https://doi.org/10.4088/JCP.09m05405blu

31. Nonacs, R. (2020, September 9). Can bright light therapy be used for the treatment of depression during pregnancy? Massachusetts General Hospital Center for Women's Mental Health, Reproductive Psychiatry Resource & Information Center. https://womensmentalhealth.org/posts/bright-light-therapy/

32. Kim, P. (2016). Human maternal brain plasticity: Adaptation to parenting, 47–58.

33. Lee, Y., Kim, K.-H., Lee, B.-H., & Kim, Y.-K. (2021). Plasma level of brain-derived neurotrophic factor (BDNF) in patients with postpartum depression. *Progress in Neuro-Psychopharmacology and Biological Psychiatry*, 109(13), 110245. https://doi.org/10.1016/j.pnpbp.2021.110245

34. Lippi, G., Mattiuzzi, C., & Sanchis-Gomar, F. (2020). Updated overview on interplay between physical exercise, neurotrophins, and cognitive function in humans. *Journal of Sport and Health Science*, 9(1), 74–81. https://doi.org/10.1016/j.jshs.2019.07.012

35. Kim, T.-W., Park, S.-S., & Park, H.-S. (2022). Effects of exercise training during advanced maternal age on the cognitive function of offspring. *International Journal of Molecular Sciences*, 23(10), 5517. https://doi.org/10.3390/ijms23105517

36. Hanson, R. (2016). *Hardwiring happiness: The new brain science of contentment, calm, and confidence.* Harmony/Rodale.

37. Melore, C. (2022, September 22). Is motherhood a glass ceiling? 46% of women say co-workers treat them unfairly for having kids. *Study Finds.* https://studyfinds.org/working-mothers-treated-unfairly-maternity-leave

38. Pawluski, J. L., et al. (2022). Less can be more: Fine tuning the maternal brain, 104475.

39. Hoekzema, E., Barba-Müller, E., Pozzobon, C., et al. (2017). Pregnancy leads to long-lasting changes in human brain structure. *Nature Neuroscience*, 20, 287–296 https://doi.org/10.1038/nn.4458

40. Parsons, C. E., Young, K. S., Petersen, M. V., Elmholdt, E-M. J., Vuust, P., Stein, A., & Kringelbach, M. L. (2017). Duration of motherhood has incremental effects on mothers' neural processing of infant vocal cues: A neuroimaging study of women. *Scientific Reports* 7, 1727. https://doi.org/10.1038/s41598-017-01776-3

41. Orchard, E. R., et al. (2023). The maternal brain is more flexible and responsive at rest: Effective connectivity of the parental caregiving network in postpartum mothers, 4719.

42. Mirin, A. A. (2021). Gender disparity in the funding of diseases by the US National Institutes of Health. *Journal of Women's Health*, 30(7), 956–963. https://doi.org/10.1089/jwh.2020.8682

43. Lakshmin, P. (2021, February 4). How society has turned its back on mothers. *The New York Times*. https://www.nytimes.com/2021/02/04/parenting/working-mom-burnout-coronavirus.html
44. Grose, J. (2021, February 4). America's Mothers Are in Crisis. *The New York Times*. https://www.nytimes.com/interactive/2021/02/04/parenting/working-moms-coronavirus.html

INDEX

degenerative processes, 21
depression. *See* postpartum depression
    and anxiety (PPDA)
desire and arousal, 66–69
dialectic/dialectical statements, 51, 65,
    157
diaphragmatic breathing, 25, 29
difficult conversations, 72–73
distorted thinking, 59–60, 97, 103–4,
    106, 114, 139, 155, 182
distraction, 6, 43–44, 85
division/depletion, 89–91
division of labor, 62–64, 118–19, 128,
    177, 183, 188, 191
divorce, 70–71
do not make things worse, 118, 120,
    165
do something different, 95
double-down method, 86–100, 192
Duke, Annie, 53, 186–87, 191
Dunn, Jancee, 61

E
effort-based reward system, 163–64
Ellison, Katherine, 151
emotions, xi, xviii
    being present, 11
    Broaden-and-Build theory, 158–59
    cognitive efficiency, 7
    emotional bank account, 72
    emotionally availability, 93, 125
    emotion-focused coping strategies,
        43–45, 80–81, 83, 85, 106
    positive emotions, 153, 158, 165
    regulation, xviii, 7, 54, 57, 153, 168,
        177
    synaptic pruning, 170–71
    transition to motherhood, 48
    upping the ante, 184
    See also mom guilt; mom rage; mom
        shame; tending to your needs first

empathy, xiv, xvi, 162, 177
engaging activities, 27–28
engaging your senses, 26, 158, 164
enriched environments, 152, 163
Epstein, Mark, 151–52
escapist shower or a bath, 82–83, 85
essentialism/responsibility, 89–91. *See
    also* roles and responsibilities
evidence-based treatments or therapies,
    xi, xvii, 39, 68, 143–45
evolution, 25, 36, 153
executive functioning, 33
exercise, 163–64
expectations, 68–69, 78, 89
experiential plasticity, 29, 151
exposures, 36, 51, 107–8, 125

F
face blanching, 43, 45, 81
Fair Labor Standards Act, 174
Fair Play (Rodsky), 62–64, 181–83
Fair Play card deck, 62, 183
Family and Medical Leave Act, 173–74
fathers, xiv, 19, 23–25, 34, 45–46, 139,
    141, 146, 152, 167, 168, 181
Feldman, Ruth, 24
fire together, wire together, 157–58, 164
5-4-3-2-1 method, 43, 45, 85
five-to-one ratio, Gottman, 71–73
flexibility, xiv, xviii, 7, 53–54, 116, 125,
    162, 168, 173–74, 182–83
Food and Drug Administration, 39
forgetfulness, x, xi, xiv, 6, 10, 150, 175
Fredrickson, Barbara, 158
fulfillment, 89, 91
functional magnetic resonance imaging
    (fMRI), xiv, 19, 77

G
general anxiety, 26